ADVANCE

GW00838608

"Wise, witty and informative... This is a book about one woman's journey to understand her own body, her own health issues and how to deal with them. On the way, she discovered a way to help all of us to recognise our own issues and has come up with a blueprint which, if we pay attention, can help all of us to take responsibility for our health... or lack of it.

Moline can be quite evangelical and every so often one must stop and take a deep breath in order digest her findings. A scientist by training, she has, over the years, through teaching, discovered how to not only make science palatable to the uninitiated (or the 'non-geeks', as she calls them), but also to make it accessible.

The whole tome is designed to hand-hold our learning process from the initial Getting Started Questionnaire, for the reader to fill in and refer to, throughout her argument. Yes, we can run to the doctor and we can take the prescription aids, but we must also look to what may be the cause of our allergies, aches and diseases, which may well be our own habits, neglect and diet.

Read carefully and take note... for Moline is at her most persuasive when she enters the regions of sleep deprivation, dehydration and ageing."

JO FOLEY, FREELANCE WRITER, EDITOR, MEDIA CONSULTANT AND INTERNATIONALLY ACKNOWLEDGED AUTHORITY ON WELLNESS AND WELLBEING.

"I feel like this book was written specially for me. I am a 'non-geek' and science bores me rigid. I am also a stage four cancer patient doing everything I can to take responsibility for my health and reverse my disease, despite being told by the conventional medical paradigm that this isn't possible.

Reboot is both brilliant and brave. The author defies much consensus 'wisdom' by unravelling the bad science behind what we are advised to eat and how we are encouraged to live. It is a shocking and sobering encounter with some essential truths about where we came from and what our bodies truly need to thrive. It seems we have created a culture that makes thriving increasingly difficult and it takes real courage to speak up for another paradigm—an ancient paradigm, indeed, one we need to remember more than reinvent.

This book has helped me understand significant contributory factors in my own disease and shown me vital actions I can take to do something about it. It is wise, witty, incredibly intelligent and easy to understand. Gerilynn's 'four horses of the chronic disease apocalypse' become four pillars upon which to build a foundation of lasting health. She has distilled years of research into this simple, game-changing volume that will undoubtedly save lives."

SOPHIE SABBAGE, AUTHOR OF *THE CANCER WHISPERER, HOW TO LET CANCER HEAL YOUR LIFE*

"I found *Reboot Yourself!* easy to read and filled with inspiring and thought-provoking information. The layout and content of the book provides clear explanations and an understanding of the necessary changes in lifestyle required to improve one's health. The need for all people to take full responsibility for their own choices is well supported by this excellent book, as it has a good balance of science, rationale, logic and Gerry's personal touch.

Overall, I totally enjoyed the process within this book of 'demystifying' the complex subject of health care. I will be recommending it to my clients and colleagues."

JOHN TINDALL, PHYSIOTHERAPIST, ACUPUNCTURIST, CHINESE MEDICINE PRACTITIONER AND FOUNDER AND DIRECTOR OF YUAN CLINIC & TRADITIONAL MEDICINE COLLEGE

"As a Healthcare professional, the subject matter of this book is very close to my own heart. We can learn through Gerry Moline's own personal journey which she shares so candidly about why so many of us are so sick, and getting sicker.

I first met Gerry at a workshop in the north of England several years ago, and I was immediately struck by her engaging presentation style, her approachability and her ability to disseminate complex material in a simple and accessible way. In her book Gerry steers a pathway for those who are lost in a quagmire of marketing and misinformation to recover optimal health, which after all *is our birthright*.

However, as Gerry rightly points out that this book is not for everybody—particularly those who are happy with the status quo, who do not yet need nor wish to venture outside the bounds of conventional healthcare, who are confident in the *system*, and are happy to blame their own sickness or increasing decrepitude on their inherited genes, and who are resigned to an inevitable and early appointment with their undertaker—this book is not for you!

'It was never my plan to write a book!'—thank goodness you did Gerry!"

CHRIS JAMES, YOGA & MEDITATION TEACHER AND OWNER OF
CHRIS JAMES MIND BODY

"What a delight. Comprehensive, fluid, written to be read, oozes with experience, and leaves you knowing you have had a conversation with a genuine, human healing force. A treasure trove of ideas, facts, intuitions and encouragements, drawing on the best of the protagonists in their fields—Becker, Batmanghelidj, Crawford, Benevista and Montagnier and many more, all presented as an entertaining story-board for the reader to absorb and become inspired and invigorated by.

There are many captivating and lyrical metaphors and turns of phrase that bring a real smile to the heart. This book will be a lighthouse for many souls floundering in their own private storms.

It should have as wide an exposure as possible."

CHRISTOPHER SCARFE, NUTRITIONAL THERAPIST AND FOUNDER
AND OWNER OF THE NUTRITION CONSULTANCY

REBOOT YOURSELF!

A NON-GEEK'S GUIDE TO REVERSING CHRONIC ILLNESS AND EARLY AGING

BY GERILYNN R. MOLINE

COPYRIGHT

Difference Press, Washington DC

Copyright © Gerilynn R. Moline, 2015

All rights reserved. No part of this book may be reproduced in any form without permission in writing from the author. Reviewers may quote brief passages in reviews.

ISBN: 978-1-68309-002-1

Library of Congress Control Number: 2015960615

DISCLAIMER

No part of this publication may be reproduced or transmitted in any form or by any means, mechanical or electronic, including photocopying or recording, or by any information storage and retrieval system, or transmitted by email without permission in writing from the author. Neither the author nor the publisher assumes any responsibility for errors, omissions, or contrary interpretations of the subject matter herein. Any perceived slight of any individual or organization is purely unintentional. Brand and product names are trademarks or registered trademarks of their respective owners.

This book contains discussions about health issues and medical problems that may be linked to our diet and environment. While the author offers some possible changes that you might make to mitigate negative environmental impacts on your health, the purpose of this book is educational and not prescriptive. It is not intended as, and is not, a substitute for professional medical advice. The author is not a physician. If you have questions about a medical problem please refer to your medical physician or primary healthcare consultant. In addition be advised that the author cannot be held responsible for medical decisions that you make as a result of reading this book, nor can the author guarantee the outcomes of any of the changes discussed in this book. Please consult your physician or healthcare professional before making any changes in your health habits or diet.

Cover Design: John Matthews

Interior Book Design: Heidi Miller

Editing: Grace Kerina

Diagrams: Gerilynn Moline

Author's photo courtesy of Joanne Logie

DEDICATION

THIS BOOK IS DEDICATED TO MY
PARENTS, BILL AND GINNY MOLINE.

*Throughout their lives they encouraged me
to read, question, explore, and make my own
unique mark on the world. Through their deaths,
they taught me much about how to face illness
with love, courage and dignity, and inspired me
to dig deep to find the work this book is based on.
I am still learning from them.*

*And to my beloved partner Hermione, without
whose unfailing love and belief in me I would
still be playing in the shadows. Your heart is
where I place my anchor.*

TABLE OF CONTENTS

1   INTRODUCTION

20   CHAPTER ONE: All I Wanted Was to Lose a
                       Little Weight

38   CHAPTER TWO: Is Your Environment
                       Flipping out Your Genes?

46   CHAPTER THREE: Mixed Messages—Our
                       'Gorilla Biscuit' Diet

82   CHAPTER FOUR: The Light of Your Life

104 CHAPTER FIVE: Personal Magnetism

118 CHAPTER SIX: A Thirst for Life

134 CHAPTER SEVEN: Blocks and Levers

146 CHAPTER EIGHT: Conclusions

153 RESOURCES

157 ACKNOWLEDGMENTS

161 ABOUT THE AUTHOR

163 THANK YOU

INTRODUCTION

"Where is the Life we have lost in living? Where is the wisdom we have lost in knowledge? Where is the knowledge we have lost in information?" T. S. ELIOT

We in the Western world (and perhaps you as an individual) are facing an unprecedented decline in health, even as life expectancy and the average standard of living are both increasing. It seems that almost every other day there is a new headline in the newspapers about some aspect of this health crisis and its current or future financial costs. Yet there does not seem to be a rational comprehensive way out of this healthcare dilemma being proposed. Instead, there is a patchwork of 'fixes' for specific issues, such as childhood obesity or dementia care. It looks more like a lot of fingers in the increasingly leaky dike holding back the rising floodwaters than any kind of cohesive plan.

I believe a new way forward is called for—one that will not be found through the lens of our current healthcare paradigm. The Western healthcare paradigm is built on key planks that severely limit our ability to see the true causes of our modern-day health crisis, at best blinding us to possible solutions and, at worst, contributing to the overall problem. For us as individuals caught up in this paradigm, we are left at the mercy of a system that can no longer have the patient or their best interests at its core. This is not to say that there are no caring doctors or that Western medicine does not have its strengths. For acute crises, I want the best that Western medicine has to offer. For chronic illness, however, Western medicine seems helpless to find a way to stem the tide.

There is a different way of looking at health and wellness, a new paradigm that opens up different questions, incorporates a new scientific understanding of how the human body functions and, therefore, points to new opportunities for healing. Even better, it is a paradigm that we as individuals can embrace and use to understand our own health issues and then take charge of our own healing. But first, it is helpful to look at a few things about our current Western medical paradigm, some foundations that it is built upon and how we got to where we are.

These are some of the elements of that paradigm:

'Doctor Knows Best'

There was a time when a key player in the medical model in the Western world was the family doctor. He or she knew all of the family members and saw them through the stages of life, sometimes from cradle to grave. A relationship of trust was built through conversation and deep knowledge of the individual, and if specialist care was needed it was arranged through that family doctor. Diagnoses were made as much through the patients' descriptions of what they were experiencing as through laboratory and testing results. There was time to hear the stories and that greatly informed the treatments given. The concept of 'doctor knows best' grew out of that relationship and the trust it engendered, but always at the heart of it was the patient. Doctors understood that listening and witnessing are integral parts of treatment.

Somehow, we got from there to where we are today, with our modern healthcare paradigm built on specialisation, managed care, and the seven-minute appointment—one in which the conversation has been lost, laboratory and test results are treated rather than the patient and the concept of 'doctor knows best' has become a result of arrogance, expediency and a system so complex that most of us have no hope of finding our way through it. So we place our lives into the hands of our physician or managed care team because we see few other choices. What has been lost is not only the relationship with the physician but also our relationship with ourselves as prime contributors in our own wellness journeys. We are at the mercy of a system in which many treatment decisions are made by administrators or government agencies or insurance companies, all bringing their own competing agendas.

I believe that the majority of doctors enter the profession because they truly want to be healers, and that they take 'first do no harm' to heart. I know and have known many of those doctors. But they, too, are affected by a system that limits their treatment options and their time with patients. The burnout rate for doctors is high.

'Better Living Through Chemistry'

Another key plank in the Western healthcare paradigm is dependence on pharmaceutical interventions for almost every known condition. I do not remember growing up with television commercials advertising prescription drugs, where a voice exhorts us to "Ask your doctor if (fill in the blank) is right for you," and then quickly rattles off a wide range of side effects, all to a background of soothing music and hopeful pictures of healthy-looking people strolling through nature. The underlying message: "Ask your doctor to give you this drug and you, too, can have a better life". The pharmaceutical solution has become so culturally engrained that when we aren't given a prescription for something to cure our complaint we feel aggrieved and somehow dismissed. This practice has had its downsides in the development of antibiotic-resistant microbes—creating the spectre of rampant, uncontrollable infections in the future—as well as the need for continuously new and different drugs to treat the side-effects of the previous drugs.

I remember seeing the piles of pills on the kitchen countertop each morning at my parents' home. I marvelled at how many there were and wondered to myself if anyone knew what the combined effect of all those chemicals was and how we ever managed for millennia without them.

When I teach my courses, I start with a flip chart filled with the names of modern-day conditions, most of which are now familiar terms, as they have become increasingly more common; and many of which are now being labelled as 'diseases of ageing', even though they rarely used to be a part of the ageing process. I then take my 'prescription pad' sticky notes, each with the name of a prescription medication on it, and paste them over each of the conditions. It drives home the picture of our pharmaceutical path to white-knuckling our way through our latter years.

'It's All in Our Genes'

Ever since Watson and Crick made their Nobel Prize–winning discovery of the structure of DNA, which led to the mapping of the entire human genome, medical science has been chasing the genetic causes of illness. Underlying this activity is an assumption that 1) most, if not all, illness has a genetic cause, and 2) if someone has a gene linked to a medical condition, they will sooner or later develop that condition, as though the gene is a predetermination. The premise: If we can find the associated gene, we can fix it with genetic engineering or develop a chemical that targets that gene. This approach predisposes a direction of health research aimed at genetic interventions.

Meanwhile, those of us who happen to have one the dreaded genetic markers—in my case, the APOE4 allele, which is associated with increased risk of Alzheimer's Disease—wait with the Sword of Damocles hanging over our heads, hoping against all hope that a new treatment comes out before our time is up.

'Managed Decline' and Other Myths of Ageing

There was a time when conditions such as diabetes and various dementias were uncommon, when even cancer and heart disease were rare. Yes, life expectancy was shorter than it is today. But, generally, people lived out their lives in relative health until biological systems began to fail in old age—unless traumatic injury or infectious disease took them at an earlier age. The benefits of modern medicine are proclaimed as we outlive our parents and grandparents, as "more people now survive cancer than die from it", as stem cell and genetic research point to new and innovative ways to treat illnesses. Yes, we are living longer. But are we living better?

The path of ageing seems to be rife with pitfalls as we make our way into our inevitable decline. We are told that, "We all get a little forgetful when we get older", that, "The old joints just give out after a while", and, "Aches and pains are just a requisite part of ageing". We're told high blood pressure and heart disease are "just a matter of time" as we get older, and we're given other messages that suggest that system failure is inevitable and we need to accept it with grace. Western medicine will help us manage that decline, usually with pharmaceutical or surgical interventions, but it rarely talks about reversal of chronic illness. People with Type 2 diabetes are told they can manage their illness for a time through dietary interventions and blood sugar–regulating medications such as Metformin, but, eventually, the pancreas will wear out and they will need insulin. We're told that joint degeneration from arthritis can be managed through high-powered anti-inflammatory and pain medications, but, eventually, the joint will no doubt need replacing. What were once relatively rare conditions are now accepted as 'normal ageing'!

How did we get here? Is this the best we can expect?

Special Interests and the Gold Standard RCT

I was a researcher for over 20 years, so I know something about how research gets funded. Money is the overriding determinant of what gets investigated and what does not. Even when political agendas determine which health issues make the front pages, research decisions ultimately come down to who will fund the programme. As such, money, more than any other factor, dictates the science agenda.

We would like to think that science is pure and impartial, above the influences of special interests, politics, ego or greed. I can tell you from experience that it is not, and that goes for medical research as well. This influence is getting a lot of publicity these days, as evidenced by stories in the popular press about the connections between the pharmaceutical companies and the medical establishment. For example, a recent newspaper story exposed the fact that NICE, the governing body in the European Union that determines which medications can be funded by government health services, is staffed by several members who have ties to major pharmaceutical companies that stand to gain through decisions made by that body.

A large part of the influence that pharmaceutical companies have over the medical research world is tied to what has now become the 'gold standard' in acceptable research protocol: the randomised controlled trial, or RCT. The RCT uses a test group and a control group to establish whether or not a particular treatment is effective or to establish whether or not a particular factor is linked to a particular condition. It has become so much the standard that other data, including anecdotal evidence or observations, are often disregarded. Thus, a whole body of information and years of human experience are dismissed as irrelevant.

RCTs take time and are expensive, so deep pockets are needed to fund them. Often, those deep pockets come with agendas that are connected to financial (or personal) gain if the results go a particular way. Let's say that a pharmaceutical company wants to run RCTs that test the effectiveness of a new drug on a particular medical condition. They're willing to make the financial investment because, if the new drug is shown to be effective, there is a large financial reward to be had by the company from putting a patent on that medication, exhorting you through TV adverts to ask your doctor to prescribe it to you, sending reps to your local surgery to make sure your doctor knows about this new treatment and generally making it a number one bestseller.

If you want to find out how effective a particular nutritional supplement or herbal remedy is for a specific health condition, however, you will be much harder pressed to find a funding source for a full-blown RCT with all its rigours. Because these substances are natural and, therefore, not patentable, there's very little money to be made from them. Often, then, what we find are case histories or anecdotal/observational evidence supporting the benefits of natural remedies—which, by the way, must be disclaimed on their packaging.

Money becomes the filter for what gets researched, what gets published in medical journals, what gets presented at medical conferences and what ultimately ends up as our treatment options. Those options become the limit of what our insurance companies will pay for. Far worse, those treatment options become the standard of care to which health professionals are held accountable. The brave souls who buck the system and refuse to practise according to this 'standard of care' can be charged with malpractice, stripped of hospital privileges, lose their license to practise or even be imprisoned. That is a strong incentive to maintain the status quo and not stray too far off the beaten path. And it's to all of our detriment.

* * *

So, here we are, those of us in the highly developed nations, with the best that medicine has to offer, the most advanced technologies, world-class practitioners and hospitals and, for most of us, good medical insurance or free health care through national healthcare systems. Yet we are getting sicker in increasing numbers at increasingly younger ages.

Obesity is reaching epidemic proportions, as are infertility, autoimmune diseases, Alzheimer's and other dementias, cancer, heart disease and more. Healthcare is a major part of our budgets, from households to governments, and we're told that the future projection of these trends is set to swamp these government budgets—as is already happening in some households.

When I talk with friends, family and clients about health, these are the kinds of statements I commonly hear:

- "There are so many confusing messages. One day they say this is good for you, and the next day they say it's bad. I don't know who or what to believe anymore."

- "I feel old before my time. I know I should be in the prime of my life, but I'm just trying to find the energy to get through the day."

- "I'm doing everything my doctor tells me to do, but I just keep getting worse. Why isn't anything helping?"

- "I've tried every diet on the planet and I still can't lose weight or keep it off. I'm told to eat less and exercise more. But I go to the gym, I eat salads, I'm hungry all the time and I *still* don't lose weight. I've been dieting all my life!"

- "My parents and grandparents had all these illnesses, so I have bad genes. It's my destiny and just a matter of time before I have them, too. I already see the signs."

- "Getting old is not for the faint-hearted. Decline is inevitable and I just have to learn to accept it with grace."

- "I would try anything, if I only knew what to try."

Perhaps you've asked some of these questions or made some of these statements yourself. I know I have, out of desperation for my own health or the health of people I care deeply about.

The Big Question: Why Are So Many of Us So Sick?

The question I hear very few people asking is, "Why is this happening?" I don't mean why is a particular person's illness happening, or even why a particular trend in illness is happening, but why are we, as a population, so sick? Why is it so much worse than 40 or 50 years ago, or even 20 years ago? Why, in spite of eating less fat since the 1970s, is there more heart disease and obesity? Why, when people are smoking less and eating more fruits and vegetables, when many chemicals like DDT have been banned, when more people are going organic, are there higher incidences of cancer? Why are so many children being diagnosed with autism, a condition that only a few decades ago was very rare? Why are more babies being born obese? What are we doing differently and what have we changed that is resulting in this explosion of chronic illness and downward-spiralling health?

Evolutionary Health: A New Paradigm

More and more now, big questions are being asked about health and healthcare. Those questions are driving the development of a new paradigm that views health and disease through the lens of our evolutionary history. This is new to our understanding, and yet in some ways it is ancient in its approach. This perspective is based on the foundation that evolution has exquisitely designed our bodies to self-heal and to function within a range of environmental conditions such that we've survived millions of years as a species—without doctors, prescriptions, medical devices, and Zimmer frames.

Starting with that premise, some interesting questions are raised. How have we survived for all this time? Have we, in recent years, changed our environmental conditions in ways that are out of alignment with how our bodies are designed to function? The human brain is so amazing that we can think up and engineer almost anything, including the climate within our homes. Have we engineered our way into disease? If so, can we do something about it? There are so many things we can eat, so many ways we can change how we live, so many choices open to us. Just because we can, does that mean we should?

This raises other questions of a more personal nature. What if your state of health is not all your fault? What if you're doing your best but you have faulty information? What if obesity and chronic illness are simply information about misalignments and what if there's a realignment that can restore health? What if there's a reset button that can reboot our systems to 'factory settings' and restore us to optimal health?

I believe that the answer to these questions is, "Yes". And that gives us reason for great hope.

An Evolutionary Path to Reversing Disease and Reclaiming Health

Biology always wins. It doesn't heed conventions or personal preferences or ethical dilemmas or religious or cultural customs. It doesn't care what your friends or neighbours think or about the latest fad or what is most convenient for you. It doesn't bend to your will. *Our biology is designed to respond to changing environmental conditions.* Many of these physical responses are adaptations to a modern environment that we now label as 'disease' or 'illness'. We can patch up the symptoms of the problem so we can continue to live the way we want to live, but that doesn't resolve the underlying conditions, and so adaptation turns into chronic illness and leads to systemic decline. *We can't bend our biology to suit our lifestyle, but we can bend our lifestyle to suit our biology.* This book will teach you how to do that.

The content of this book incorporates the results of leading-edge research into the effects of various environmental and dietary factors on our physiology that paint a new picture of how our bodies respond to our environment. The result is a framework that provides a new lens for viewing health and wellbeing to make sense of what we're seeing in current health trends. Along with this framework are guidelines for making lifestyle changes that can halt and even reverse a downward spiral into chronic illness and early ageing. You will learn how to begin to take charge of your own health and wellbeing, become your own best health advocate and make sense of so many mixed messages about healthy living. Finally, you will find guidance about how to handle the internal and external blocks that can get in the way of making the changes you know you want to make.

I have walked this path myself, as have others I know, and I can attest to the power of this new way of living. My path will not be your path exactly, as each path is individual, but I will show you how to begin to find yours. As a wise teacher told me in reference to my future health, "Nothing is written in stone" and "It's never too late to start". That was a message of hope in a sea of messages about the inevitability and predetermination of my decline, and I have been proving that wise teacher right ever since.

The goal of this book is to liberate you to reclaim the vitality that is your birthright by design.

How to Use This Book

The content of this book is derived from years of researching what is being discovered outside of the Western healthcare model and that challenges conventional wisdom about diet and nutrition and, in fact, our fundamental understanding about how the human body works. It incorporates my background as a registered nurse, a scientific researcher, a Functional Diagnostic Nutrition® practitioner and a transformational trainer and coach, as well as my experience of finding my way back into vitality and reversing my own chronic illness.

I am a scientist at heart, with a deep background in biology and physics. I am also a big-picture person who loves to connect the dots. In the science world, there are 'generalists' and 'specialists'. Generalists have knowledge in several areas and tend to find multidisciplinary solutions to problems. Specialists, on the other hand, make it their mission to know as much as possible about their particular area of expertise. We need both. The latter is much like modern medicine, which has become more and more specialised and compartmentalised in its approach. I fall into the former category. I am a generalist. I absorb apparently disparate bits of information and then connect the dots into a coherent picture of how things interrelate. This is also what I believe modern-day medicine and medical research are missing and why our approach to both (as well as our experience of them) is often patchy and ultimately fails to turn the tide of chronic illness. There are shining stars in the healthcare field who are knitting those patches of insight and hope together into a quilt. They are my teachers, lighting the way into this new paradigm, and I will tell you about them.

I am also a teacher. My great joy is to distil information and then translate it into a picture that makes sense to others. I do this type of translation for my workshop participants and I personalise its application with my coaching clients. I may like to know the minutiae about quantum biology and how Einstein's theories govern mitochondrial processes, but most of my clients and, I daresay, readers of this book will not. Rest assured, that type of knowledge is not needed in order to reclaim your vitality!

This book is based on hard science, but distilled into a more generally understandable message. My aim is to make that understanding accessible to most people, because it is through understanding that we can find our way through the fog of mixed messages and become empowered to make informed decisions on our own behalf.

This book is *not* the whole story, but is a comprehensive starting place for building knowledge and taking action. By the end of it, you will know more than most people on the planet about how our bodies really work, and you will have the foundation for making choices that will improve your health immediately and in the longer term. For those of you who do want to delve more deeply, I've provided a list of resources at the end of the book to give you a leg up in your search.

In the next chapter, I'll tell you how I stumbled onto this path of recovery at a most unlikely time of my life, and how I discovered through my own research and healing that most of my (and our) understanding about how we function has been built on erroneous information and a faulty foundation.

In subsequent chapters, I'll lay out four key areas in which your modern-day lifestyle is likely to be significantly impacting your health in ways that you don't even suspect, and tell you about some specific things you can to do mitigate those effects in order to bring your environment into alignment with how your body best functions and heals. Finally, I include a chapter on the kinds of things that may trip you up as you begin to take steps on your journey into wellness, how you might handle them and how to find allies on your quest.

I will teach you how to be an evolutionary detective—how to find misalignments in your environment, how to identify interventions you can make and how to monitor the results so you have data about yourself and about what works for you. You will become the expert in you.

A word of caution: This material is intended solely for educational purposes, and is not intended to replace the advice of your current healthcare programme or practitioner. I share the results of my evolutionary sleuthing with my practitioner and encourage you to share your findings with yours. In Chapter Seven I talk about how to get your healthcare practitioner into partnership with you so that you can merge the best of the conventional and nonconventional approaches.

The 'Get Started' Questionnaire

It is always helpful when embarking on a journey to know where your starting point is. Because you will be 'researching' yourself, you will need some data about how things are now as a baseline to measure your progress against. This will allow you to keep track of the effects of the changes you make along the way. It will also guide you to your next steps and become your recipe for 'the proof in the pudding', metaphorically speaking—your proof that aligning yourself with how nature designed you is your ticket to health.

To get you started with this process, you can download and fill out a 'Get Started' Questionnaire from my website (evolutionaryreboot.com/get-started-questionnaire).

Make copies of the questionnaire so you can use it here at the beginning—filling the questionnaire out every day for a week—to give yourself a good set of baseline data. Then refer to it as you read through the chapters of the book, noticing what your answers reveal about you and your environment. Filling out additional copies of the questionnaire as you begin to implement changes will help you gather additional data and track the impact of those changes. In particular, pay attention to the questions that address your level of energy and sense of wellbeing. This journey is not only about halting or reversing disease—it's about reclaiming your vitality!

CHAPTER ONE

All I Wanted Was to Lose a Little Weight

"Look deep, deep into nature,and then you will understand everything better." ALBERT EINSTEIN

Actually, I wanted more than that when I started out, but I had given up on a future of robust health. In fact, when I met my partner I came with a list of health warnings: diabetes, heart disease, degenerative arthritis, cancers of all kinds and the dreaded Alzheimer's. "I have bad genes", I said, "and these diseases are my likely future. Just want you to know what you're signing up for".

I have struggled on and off, mostly on, with weight all my life. You name a diet or a weight-loss remedy and I have probably tried it. I did manage some stretches of time where the weight stayed off for a while, like when I was training for a marathon or heavily involved in sport, but most of the time it just came back, with a little more for good measure. Of course, I took that as a very personal failure and evidence of some weakness of will at my core.

If that were all there was to my history, then I wouldn't be writing this book. I might still be googling my way through those ads that start out with "Lose 10 pounds in 5 days!" and then make you listen through 20 minutes of promises and testimonials before you get to the "Money Back Guarantee Special Offer" bottles of some Amazonian root used for thousands of years by the skinny jungle tribes and only recently discovered by the Western explorers and brought to you exclusively by their company for a limited time only while supplies last... before buying the product and finding out, because you didn't read the small print, that you are automatically billed at the ultra-high normal price once the trial period ends and, by the time you realize that, you're a month into the automatic billing and it takes you another two weeks to get the auto-payments cancelled and, by the way, the stuff doesn't work anyway. Whew! Yes, if you're laughing, then I know you may have done this, too.

My story might have been comic, sad, run-of-the-mill even. I might have lost the same weight over again many more times before I found my ticket to a healthier, more vibrant future. For that, things had to get worse. A lot worse.

When I was in my forties, I started having "glitches", times when I would forget well-known pieces of information—the names of acquaintances or even good friends, my phone number, information I had just read, common vocabulary, and more. I once found myself driving home, via a route I had driven countless times before, and getting confused at one of the road junctions. For a brief, horrifying moment I didn't know where I was. Occasionally, I would have difficulty comprehending the material I was reading and would have to read it over again, sometimes more than once. I might pick up a novel that I hadn't gotten to yet and get one or two chapters into it, only to discover that I had actually read it before but had only a hazy recollection of the story.

I call those incidences 'glitches' because they were episodic, coming and going without warning and without any identifiable pattern. In between glitches I functioned at a very high level. I was a researcher at a U.S. Government laboratory, having completed masters and doctoral degrees in geophysics and hydrogeology. My work required taking in and absorbing vast amounts of information, making sense of it, and finding creative solutions to environmental problems. I lived by my intellect, defined myself by it, even, and had built a research programme, published papers, and presented at international conferences—all while becoming a master at finding ways to compensate, cover, and hide the glitches and lapses.

I developed strategies like writing down key information before making phone calls, lest I get caught out not remembering something like my own phone number. And I took it all as a sign that I was starting to travel down a predestined road to early-onset dementia, like my mother, her sisters, and her mother before her had. The ladies in my family had not fared well in their later years. My mother was just 60 when I first experienced her telling me the same story again five minutes after she had first told it to me. I suspect that she, too, had been compensating for many years before that.

I underwent neuropsychological testing after the glitches started, self-paid and in secret, to try to find an answer or some confirmation that I was on that same path. I performed well on the tests—spectacularly, in fact—except for experiencing one obvious glitch in the midst of them. Had the neurologist not observed me having a glitch, he wouldn't have known what I was describing. But he did see it and he agreed that it was abnormal. The test results didn't show anything untoward because, as he described it, I was "too high-functioning". The only thing I could do, he said, was re-test every five years or so and wait to see if things got worse. They did.

Scroll forward another decade. I was by then living in the UK, having left the research world and transitioned into doing transformational training and consulting with a company based in London. The glitches were more frequent, but my compensation skills were honed to a fine art and I had no trouble performing at a high level. My parents' health had been going downhill for some time, though, in a process that was heart-breaking to watch. In spite of the best that medicine had to offer and full insurance coverage, the list of their chronic conditions seemed to keep piling up: high blood pressure, atherosclerosis, Type-2 diabetes, osteoarthritis, osteoporosis, obesity, kidney failure, colon cancer, breast cancer, dementia. In spite of a background in nursing (my first career), I felt helpless to know what to suggest, and frightened that I was looking at my own body's future.

Then, in the summer of 2007, my father died suddenly, my mother needed to be placed in care, we lost the family home, my brother became gravely ill and was put into intensive care, my beloved teacher died, and a relationship ended—all within the space of less than 3 months. I experienced each of those events as body blows and, in a sense, they were. My health took a steep dive during that time, and continued to decline for years. By Christmas of that year, my clothes were falling off me, most of the major joints of my body ached, I was so weak when I went home to visit that I had to have my sister-in-law help lift my suitcase up two little steps, I literally fell asleep on my dinner, I felt like my brain was in a fog half the time and I had to drag myself up by my bootstraps in the morning. I would wake myself up several times a night when just the act of turning over caused intense pain.

That was when I first fully engaged with the Western medical system as a consumer. Previously, I had been on the other side, as a giver of care, and had prided myself on the fact that I had been so healthy all my life—outside of that little issue of the weight and that other little issue of the glitches, of course.

First there were blood tests, which showed nothing other than high inflammatory markers, at levels where they say there is "significant underlying pathology". Later, I would find out that they also showed low thyroid function, but they somehow missed telling me that. The recommended treatment was a course of high-powered anti-inflammatory drugs that did little other than take the edge off of the pain. Oh, and which required periodic liver tests and prescription changes to keep the drugs from destroying my liver. Then I was referred to a rheumatologist, who took more blood tests and determined that my thyroid function was low but my lab results were "not bad enough yet" to treat it. If falling asleep in my mashed potatoes wasn't "bad enough yet", I shuddered to think how bad it had to get.

In the end, I spent two and a half years being monitored and tested in every conceivable way, each time getting more blood drawn, each time being told my inflammatory markers were still high, each time being told the doctors couldn't figure out what was going on but to come back in a couple of months, each time being passed on to a different doctor at the clinic and having to tell them the story from the beginning when they said, "So what brings you here today?" as if there was nothing written in my chart. I stopped the anti-inflammatory drugs myself out of fear for my liver and stomach and the fact that they did little good.

Meanwhile, I was still working full-time, travelling nearly every week within the UK and internationally to deliver residential trainings, and flying back and forth to the US to spend time with my mother until she, too, died. By that time, something had shifted and I was piling on the weight again, my sleep was shredded, and I would wake in the night drenched in sweat. I felt much older than my years and often looked it, too.

I found a doctor who actually listened to the symptoms I was describing, decided it was indeed bad enough and prescribed thyroid medication, which did help a bit. When the rheumatologist said he didn't know what was going on and that I should just return in a year to be tested again, I knew they had given up on me and that I was on my own with my illness, whatever it was. So I gave up on them and, in resigning myself to early ageing, chronic pain, and cognitive decline, gave up on myself as well, along with a future that included health and vitality.

Two key things happened then that turned the tide for me. The first was being introduced to a woman who practices Traditional Chinese Medicine and acupuncture. Her methods did have a beneficial effect on the pain and low energy, but the biggest change she helped me with was a shift in my fear of dementia. I stopped believing that it was a sure bet and made peace with it as only a possible outcome.

After two years of Traditional Chinese Medicine treatment, I was ready again to tackle the weight issue. I was given a copy of Tim Ferriss' book *The Four-Hour Body* and I started to follow his dietary plan for body recomposition. All I really wanted was to lose a little weight.

What happened was that within the first week and a half of following Ferriss' plan, not only did I lose a few pounds and inches, my sleep became deep and restful, I stopped sweating in the night, my joint pain went away, I woke feeling refreshed and energised, and my inflammatory markers began to drop. Changing my diet began to do what two and a half years of medical treatment had failed to do.

I am a scientist. I needed to know why.

The second key thing that happened was that I became a researcher again. I had taken a short sabbatical from work and I decided to use the resulting free time to delve into what was happening with my body and why it was responding the way it was to a dietary changes I'd made. I was a researcher by profession, so I knew how to research a problem. I had previously been a nurse, so I knew something about how the human body works. And I had time. So I started reading everything I could get my hands on in the field of nutrition, which led me to the whole ancestral health movement, which led me to websites and blogs and PubMed articles and more books. I was crunching through two to three books a week, plus countless website materials, and it was like that *Twilight Zone* episode where the guy sticks his head through a soft spot in the wall and sees a whole new reality on the other side. Everything I had learned about health and nutrition had been built on shaky or incomplete science, and it all fell apart like a house of cards.

I went after the answer to the question, "Why is all this chronic disease happening—not just with me and my parents, but with skyrocketing numbers of people in the developed world?" Thus began four years of immersion into a field of study which you would be hard-pressed to find taught in any kind of comprehensive programme: evolutionary health and nutrition. If I'd found such a programme, I would have signed up in a heartbeat, but there isn't yet one in existence that goes to the heart of the quantum nature of how our bodies function in connection with and in response to our environment. The relationship between our human bodies and the environment was designed through evolutionary changes over millions of years.

There is now more of a focus on ancestral diets, which is at the heart of the Paleo Diet and which is the topic of numerous books and websites. That was where my search started and how my own interventions began. I came to understand that the diet I was following from Ferriss' book was mostly a paleo template and that it was having a positive effect on my health not only because of *what* I was eating but also *when* I was eating. Through my research, I stumbled onto the website of a brilliant American neurosurgeon, Dr. Jack Kruse, who has been knitting the pieces of the puzzle into a comprehensive understanding of human physiology he aptly calls 'The Quilt'. His website (jackkruse.com) is not for sissies. If you're looking for a simple to-do list you won't find it there. What you will find is a series of blogs and webinars that will teach you about the pieces of The Quilt with all of their depth and complexity, will show you how we are inextricably linked to the earth and the cosmos, and will provide concrete answers to the questions "Why is this happening?", "How are we causing our own demise?", and "What can we do about it?"

Dr. Kruse's mission is to educate, and so his materials point to the sources of the information, which has informed my own search. I go to the source. He does not want followers. He wants to develop thinkers who will pave a new way forward. Perhaps his most important influence on me personally was when he told me, in response to a question I raised on his site about dementia, that, "Nothing is written in stone" and "It's never too late to start". That, coming from a neurosurgeon with his depth of knowledge, gave me hope for a healthy future that I had stopped daring to dream of. I have been repairing my health ever since, and proving him right.

The Challenge of the Well-Meaning and Conventionally Indoctrinated

Overcoming the pull of conventional wisdom on my path to wellness has been a bit like trying to swim away from the suction of a sinking ship. Picture the scene in the movie *Titanic* where Jack and Rose, the protagonists and unfortunate passengers, fight their way to the surface as the ship disappears beneath the waves. I know my own body better than anyone else, including my doctors, and yet it has been an upward battle to climb into the fresh air and lay claim to that knowledge and to trust it in the face of well-meaning family, friends and health professionals who purport to know better than I what I am experiencing and what is real for me.

Conventional wisdom is a powerful force that expresses itself in sentences that begin with "They say that..." and "Everyone knows that..." and in slogans like "Five a day" and

"No pain, no gain". Conventional wisdom is the basis for our dietary choices, for the products we consume, for the environments we create in our homes, and for the way we structure our lives. It is what we fall back on as the foundation that dictates our health habits or targets. It drives government health policies, advertising revenues, and billions of dollars and pounds worth of product development. You may not know the strength of conventional wisdom when you're floating in the soup with everyone else, but you will soon discover it as you try to swim your way up and out of the bowl.

In this climate, it has been difficult to find true allies in my quest for health. I was lucky enough to find an NHS doctor who would work with me within the limitations of what the NHS (UK's National Health Service) could offer. The rest I had to find and fund myself, such as lab tests to measure things the NHS did not deem important enough to measure. I found names and data for what was happening to me—fibromyalgia, adrenal stress, Hashimoto's thyroiditis, metabolic syndrome, and leptin resistance. My hormone panel was trashed, my adrenal glands were struggling to keep up and losing, my immune system was on high alert, and my body was attacking itself. No one tested for these things because such tests are not part of the conventional approach. I needed those results, though, because finding the way out requires first knowing where you are.

Ultimately, I needed to create my own path to restoring my health. Because I took the time and made the effort to learn about and trust my own body, I could use my body's responses to validate changes I made in my diet and my environment. I gathered data on myself in the way I used to gather data in my research lab, and then used that data to inform the next steps. I was and still am my own unique, individual experiment.

My health is not fully optimal yet. Chronologically, I am four years older than I was when I started. Physiologically, I am probably ten years younger. I have good energy throughout the days and I think more clearly. I no longer ache, my inflammatory markers are down, and I sleep well almost all of the time (except when I do silly things that I know will disrupt my sleep). I have vitality—that zest for life I remember having as a child. I wake up looking forward to the day. Best of all, I no longer look at a future of continual decline, believing the best years are behind me and feeling helpless to stem the tide. I may not be able to control all of what will happen to me, but I know I have the ability to significantly impact the direction my health is headed. I know, because I already have. I am a lifelong student of myself and I will be a lifelong student of how our magnificent bodies function, educating myself as new research becomes available and this new paradigm of evolutionary health unfolds.

An Unlikely Author

It was never my plan to write a book. In fact, as I have begun to build an educational business around evolutionary health over the past few years, when people have asked me if I've written a book I've replied that, "We don't need another book. People need to know about the books that are already out there." The information is all there for the taking for those who are willing to look, read and explore. But my response ignored the fact that I've spent years accumulating the knowledge that is "out there," through a deep, intensive and professionally experienced dive, and that much of the most important bits are found at a deep scientific level that many people are not interested in pursuing. I am, without a doubt, a geek, and so I soak up the minutiae of quantum biology. The majority of the people I know are not geeks, so I'm writing this book to share what I've learned with people like them.

I started my business because I want people to know what I and others have discovered—that early ageing and chronic degenerative diseases are not a given. I want people to know that they have within their grasp the ability to change their environment in ways that will allow them to regain their health and vitality, that many chronic conditions are reversible, that it is possible to reboot the body's systems.

I've been haunted by the thought that I might have been able to make a significant impact on my parents' health if only I had known then what I came to know through my research. People within and outside of the modern healthcare system tell me that it will take at least 15 to 20 years for much of what has been discovered to find its way into that system, because of our society's deep investment in the current paradigm of conventional wisdom. I can't afford to wait that long, and I know that there are others who can't or don't want to either.

In my workshops and coaching sessions, I work with people who want to improve their health, who have tried many things without success and who are invested in making positive changes—if they only knew what to change. I don't prescribe, I don't diagnose and I don't hand out how-to lists. Instead, I teach my clients how to make changes based on evolutionary principles and how to tailor those changes to their own circumstances. I distil the science into a form that can be grasped by non-scientists, in order to teach a framework for making changes and evaluating the results. I support my clients in making changes in stages in order to take charge of their recovery and become the architects of their own healthier future.

This book has the same purpose. It is drawn from the material I include in my workshops and coaching sessions. It is not the whole story, by any means, but it does describe an approach that is based on evolutionary principles and that has been applied with good results. Not everyone will want to go outside the bounds of the conventional healthcare model to get well. That's absolutely okay—we each have to choose our own path. But if you're not willing to go outside the bounds of convention, then this book is probably not for you. Others of you will want health badly enough to do whatever it takes, even if it means going against conventional wisdom. If that's you and you want your health back—if only you knew where to begin—this book is for you.

My Approach: The Four Horsemen of the Chronic Illness Apocalypse

In this book I discuss four key areas in which we have so significantly altered our environment and the way we live that we are out of alignment with how our bodies were designed over millions of years of evolution to function. I will tell you how these misalignments are manifesting in the majority of the chronic illnesses we're experiencing today, and I will suggest some changes you can make to begin to restore your body to its optimal functioning. I call these key areas the Four Horsemen of the Chronic Illness Apocalypse because a misalignment in any one of them will undermine the body's ability to heal itself and to function optimally, ultimately leading to chronic illness and early ageing. The four areas are:

- Diet

- Light

- Electromagnetism

- Water

In the chapter, 'Our Gorilla Biscuit Diet', I start with topic of diet, not because it is the most important factor—it's not—but because it's the common starting point for many of the clients I see, just as it was for me. Intractable weight gain and digestive disorders are often the things that leave people desperately searching for help, even though they don't know those issues are merely symptoms of the body responding to a bad environment (which includes the food we put into our mouths). I also start with diet because changes in diet can bring some immediate results, including the restoration of energy. When people begin to feel better, they're motivated to make other changes, and they have more physical resources for doing so. Such changes can restore other functions at a fundamental level.

In the chapter called 'The Light of Your Life', I begin to delve more deeply into something called 'circadian biology' and the importance of the body's ability to tell time. I look at how we evolved within light and dark cycles, and unveil some of the mysteries about what happens when we sleep—and when we don't. If you have never been a sun-worshipper before, you may become one once you know how sunlight powers the very life within us as undeniably as it powers the plants around us. This may be the most important thing you learn about how the body works and how our modern environment causes havoc at the most fundamental levels of our physiology.

In the chapter on 'Personal Magnetism' we'll explore the electrical nature of our bodies—how the body communicates with itself to initiate healing, and the nature of our built-in GPS system, which receives important signals from our environments. This leads to an understanding of how modern technology is disrupting our circuit boards, shorting out our systems, and what we can do about it.

In the final chapter of the key areas for realignment, 'A Thirst For Life', we'll explore the incredibly important role water plays in making our systems function, and why you cannot drink your way into being fully hydrated in our technological world. This chapter ties together threads from the previous chapters and shows how some ancient treatment methodologies may turn out to have some very solid science at their foundation.

I encourage you to read those four key chapters in order, as each one builds on the understanding of the previous ones.

I hope that you enjoy what you read and that it stimulates your curiosity and brings you to a new understanding about what makes you tick at the most basic levels.

If you're struggling with health issues, my wish is that as you read through this book you find fresh hope and a way to begin to move in the direction of restored health and vitality. Remember, as a wise man once told me, nothing is written in stone and it's never too late to start.

CHAPTER TWO

Is Your Environment Flipping out Your Genes?

"Illnesses do not come upon us out of the blue. They are developed from small daily sins against Nature. When enough sins have accumulated, illnesses will suddenly appear." HIPPOCRATES

Humans are the only mammals capable of re-engineering their environment (and the environments of countless other species as a consequence). For hundreds of thousands of years, humans adapted to environmental conditions ranging from equatorial tropics to high-latitude permafrost, and everything in between. As a species, we've weathered seasonal changes, ice ages, abundance, and scarcity.

These days, we don't adapt to environmental changes, we change our environment—through the marvels of central heating and air conditioning, modern lighting, amply protective wardrobes and global food supply chains—or we escape altogether, thanks to transport that can take us from one environment to another within hours. Nowadays, we are effectively removed from direct connection to the outside environment, because we create indoor environments that remain relatively constant (and comfortable) year-round. We can even stack ourselves vertically to live densely clustered on top of each other in comfort.

Many species are restricted to very narrow environmental conditions—so narrow, in fact, that the species may only be found in one small geographic location. Their sensitivity to environmental conditions is the reason certain species, such as frogs, are used by scientists as indicators—like the canary in the coalmine—of the effects of climate change. One might wonder, then, what gave humans the ability to adapt to such diverse, changing environments throughout our evolutionary history. It turns out that the answer is in our genes, but not in the way you might expect. Take a deep breath now, because I'm about to launch into a bit of science in order to set the stage for understanding how we got into the health pickle we find ourselves in, and so we can figure out how to get out of it.

Back in the 1800s, a monk by the name of Gregor Mendel filled in the time between his devotions to God by playing around with pea plants. He discovered that by cross-pollinating different species of peas he could produce predictable variations, thus launching what would become the field of science known as 'genetics'.

Most of us learned in introductory biology classes that our genes (the building blocks of our DNA) are located in the nucleus of each cell, that they are lodged within of pairs of chromosomes (half from each parent), and that they control such characteristics as eye colour and blood type.

Scientists came to believe that many things are 'hard-wired' into our genes, controlling physiological characteristics, predispositions to certain illnesses and possibly even our behaviour and how we think.

That launched a whole area of research in which investigations have focused on issues such as whether certain characteristics are controlled by 'nature or nurture', and whether or not there are genes that can be linked to things like criminal behaviour. Other research, such as the effects of being exposed to ionising radiation and carcinogenic chemicals, has shown that damage to our chromosomes, usually during cell division, can result in cancers and other diseases.

Our genes have been viewed as master controllers of our makeup and our functioning, and research has become ever more focused on the development of gene therapies that can alter how particular genes function, in order to halt or prevent disease. There's also the belief that our genes have evolved over time, thus allowing humans to survive changes in the environment over time.

What is puzzling about this whole picture of how our genes work is that the human genome has changed very little from that of our ancestors 200,000 years ago. Yes, there are variations between individuals that give us our unique characteristics, but the basic structure of the human genome is common to all of us and, apparently, to our distant ancestors as well. Not much has fundamentally changed in our DNA over the course of many thousands of generations. However, two discoveries about the human genome have turned our earlier understanding of human genetics on its head.

The first discovery was that we actually have two sets of genes—one set that's in each cell's nucleus, and which we got from both parents, and a second set found in our mitochondria—the microscopic engines within each of our cells that convert the food we eat into energy to fuel our bodies. Mitochondrial DNA (as opposed to nuclear DNA) is inherited solely from our mothers, handed down through each generation. It controls, among other things, our metabolic processes and two essential biological programmes: *autophagy,* which allows our bodies to repair or replace damaged proteins, and *apoptosis,* which limits cell growth by programmed death. If you think of the unrestrained growth of damaged cells that occurs with the development of cancerous tumours, you can appreciate the significance of this discovery.

Because changes to this DNA happen so infrequently, scientists can now use our mitochondrial DNA to trace our lineage back to its origins. In the book *The Seven Daughters of Eve*, Bryan Sykes traces the whole of the human population back to seven original mothers, allowing anthropologists to map out the patterns of human migration from our East African origins.

If the basic structure of our human genome has changed so little for at least the past 200,000 years and our mitochondrial DNA has changed few enough times that it allows us to trace back to our origins, how have we managed to adapt to such widely varying environmental conditions? The answer lies in the second big discovery. It turns out that most of our genes are not 'fixed' after all, but behave differently in different environmental conditions. Even further, each gene can dictate the production of not just one protein, as originally thought, but several different proteins, depending on the environmental signals received. This ability of genes to respond to environmental changes is known as 'epigenetics', which literally means 'above genetics'. It turns out that our genes are not so much master controllers as master responders.

It would help to have a definition of 'epigenetics', so here is one from Wikipedia (with my emphasis added via italics): "It refers to functionally relevant modifications to the genome that do not involve a change in the nucleotide sequence.... These changes may remain through cell divisions for the remainder of the cell's life *and may also last for multiple generations*. However, there is no change in the underlying DNA sequence of the organism; instead, *non-genetic factors cause the organism's genes to behave (or 'express themselves') differently.*"

Here's the non-scientific interpretation: Although some genes—whether they're found in mitochondrial DNA or nuclear DNA—are hard-wired, most have switches that allow them to flip on and off, depending on the person's internal and external environments. That is what allows us our great adaptability. It also means that the effects of environmental conditions on the body are passed on to off-spring from the mother and from her mother before her. This is a survival mechanism that allows the mother to 'set the switches' for her unborn baby in order to maximise her offspring's survival under the existing conditions.

It makes sense that the characteristics that most determine our ability to adapt to environmental conditions are controlled by our mitochondrial DNA, inherited from our mothers. It also explains why the females of our species are more sensitive to environmental changes and have greater reactions to misalignments. If you ladies reading this have ever grumbled about the fact that men seem to be able to get away with a lot more 'abuse' of the body, that weight loss diets seem to work on them so much more quickly when all we women have to do is think about a slice of chocolate cake and we can feel our waistbands tightening... you can blame it on our genes. An analogy I once heard was that the balance beam men walk along is three feet wide (they could practically stagger along it in a drunken stupor), but for women it's more like three inches wide (requiring a delicate tiptoe and focused attention). We women were designed by evolution to protect the next generation and, therefore, to sensitively read environmental cues.

This new understanding of the role of genetics in how we function within our environment leads to a whole new way of looking at chronic illnesses, which are sometimes referred to as 'Neolithic diseases' because they have modern-day origins (as opposed to 'Paleolithic', or ancient origins). Instead of being the result of pre-programmed 'bad' genes, many, if not most, of our modern-day illnesses can be seen as adaptations to a bad environment. When I say 'bad environment', I'm not talking about the global warming issue that we've all heard about, but something much more up close and personal, which I will reveal in the remaining chapters.

The good news is that because these genetic changes are not hard-wired they can possibly be reversed, thus rebooting our physical systems back to factory settings. The bad news is that we need to change our environment in order to change the way our body is responding. That doesn't mean going back to living in caves and hunting and foraging for food without any modern conveniences. But it does require each of us to evaluate the environment we've created around us and to make informed and discerning choices about how much we're willing to change in order to reclaim our health and vitality. From an epigenetic standpoint, it appears that we can't always have our cake and eat it, too.

In her book *The Sixth Extinction*, Elizabeth Kolbert describes how life on Earth has experienced five great extinction events during which as much as 90% of all living species disappeared suddenly and dramatically (in geologic terms), usually due to a cataclysmic event, such as the asteroid impact that killed off the dinosaurs. She presents evidence that strongly suggests we're in the midst of a sixth extinction event, one that's unfolding significantly more rapidly than any of the previous events, and one that we're creating as a result of the way we're impacting not only our local environments but our global environment as well.

Clearly, the way we're changing our environment in the Western world is having an impact on the world as a whole, our health as individuals, and the health of our offspring— as epigenetics dictates. This explains why we're seeing Neolithic diseases occurring not only in greater frequency with each generation, but at younger ages. Type 2 diabetes used to be considered an age-related disease. Now the incidence in children is rising. A 3-year-old in the United States was recently diagnosed with Type 2 diabetes—the youngest person to date to receive this diagnosis.

The connection between environment and chronic illness is undeniable when we increasingly see people in developing countries begin to succumb to the same pattern of rising incidences of chronic disease in the wake of the exportation of Western diets and technology. We don't need randomised controlled trials to prove this connection. We have centuries of observation.

When we understand how our bodies were designed to respond to environmental changes, we're pointed toward what we need to do to reverse the effects.

What elements of our environment have we changed in ways that are contributing to our individual and collective demise? How are those changes flipping our switches? And what can we do about it? Read on to find out.

CHAPTER THREE

Mixed Messages—Our 'Gorilla Biscuit' Diet

"The doctor of the future will no longer treat the human frame with drugs, but rather will cure and prevent disease with nutrition." **THOMAS EDISON**

If we're looking for evolutionary misalignments that might be creating our downward-spiralling health as a species, a good place to start is with our diet, as food is one of the ways our bodies come into direct contact with our environment.

Food is energy, that much we know. What most of us don't know is that food is also information—information about the abundance and types of energy available to us, about what season it is, about the lengths of days, about how warm or cool it is. Food's energy is matched to the environment in which it is produced, whether it's from plant or animal sources. That information is coded into the sub-atomic particles known as electrons that are contained within the food's atomic structure.

When I say that "food is information" I don't mean in a conscious sense, like knowing that asparagus and strawberries are spring crops here in the UK or that the lambing season comes at a certain time of year so you know the best time to buy a fresh Sunday roast. What I mean is that food contains energetic information that's transmitted from the electrons it contains directly to the mitochondria in our cells. That energy is utilised to power our bodies through a process called 'electron chain transport'. Evolution has exquisitely designed us with the capacity to read that coded information and adjust our systems accordingly. You don't have to understand the nuances of subatomic particle physics to grasp what this means. I'll give you a metaphor.

When I lived in the northeastern part of the U.S., I heated my home with a wood-burning stove. But not all wood burns the same, as I discovered. Pine burns hot and quick, while harder woods, such as oak, burn cooler and more slowly. If I wanted fast heat I would start the fire with pine then put a big piece of oak in the stove to keep the fire burning through the night. Obviously, we don't burn our food in tiny, cellular woodstoves (although those who measure the energy in food as calories seem to think so!), but this is a useful metaphor for thinking about how certain foods burn hotter than others. In my woodstove, the fuel I gave it released energy as heat. In my mitochondria, the fuel I give my body as food releases energy as electrons.

Where does the energy in food come from? Ultimately, it comes from sunlight that was captured by the plants we eat or by the plants that were eaten by the animals we eat. We literally eat sunlight. Those of us living nearer the poles know that that the intensity of sunlight varies throughout the year and across the globe. That's why every outdoor green space in London is mobbed by fishbelly-white bodies the minute the sun begins to show the least bit of warmth, and why we hightail it to more equatorial climes to escape the grey winter days.

It turns out that we do more than eat sunlight (more about that in the next chapter), but the main thing to know for now is that *the energy in our foods is a reflection of the energy of the environment in which the food was formed.* Thus, that banana from Honduras is going to have a different electron signal than that strawberry from the southeast of England. One way of creating an environmental mismatch is to live in one environment and consume foods from a completely different environment. That sends mixed messages to our bodies.

If we now zoom out from the subatomic level (whew!) to a more macroscopic view, we see other mismatches, ways we're living that don't align with our bodies' evolutionary design. These misalignments cause modern-day illnesses as our bodies try to adapt to the materials and messages they're receiving through our food. It appears that *what* we eat and the timing of *when* we eat matter greatly.

The Paleo Platter

First of all, how do we know what we're supposed to be eating? Diet has been the topic of some of the biggest and most contentious health debates over the past five or six decades. Food is big business. Decisions about what constitutes a healthy diet in our Western culture affect growers, manufacturers, marketers, retailers and consumers. The food we consume today—ready meals, highly processed ingredients and loads of chemical additives—bears little resemblance to what was on the tables of our grandparents or great-grandparents, and resembles even less what our hunter-gatherer ancestors consumed.

A look through the evolutionary lens indicates that our ancestral diet was based primarily on whatever could be hunted, trapped or gathered on land or fished from the waters. Many of our early ancestors were nomadic, moving with the seasons to follow food sources such as migrating game.

There are many disagreements about what constituted our ancestral diet, about whether it was meat-based or plant-based (which often has the Paleo Diet crowd pitted against the vegan crowd), and about what the various macronutrient ratios were. The impetus for much of this debate has at its heart a recognition that our modern diet is contributing to our current health crises and that if we were to return to the diet of our ancestors it would resolve some of those issues. To say that the debate is coloured by vested interests, egos, personalities, monetary gain and dogma is not an overstatement. It is beyond the focus of this book to go into all the details of that debate, nor is it necessary to fully define what the ancestral diet was in order to understand the impacts from how it has changed.

For the moment, let us take as given that the ancestral diet varied by geography, seasons and climate cycles, according to food availability at any given time and place. Our ancestors ate what was available, when and where it naturally occurred.

One thing that's certain is that we've evolved from the dominantly plant-based diet of our primate cousins, the apes. Our physiology evolved away from the primate body in some very significant ways. Firstly, our gut shortened, which signals a change to a more nutrient-dense diet that includes higher percentages of animal fat and protein. Apes have a long section of lower intestine in which bacteria break down plant fibres and convert them into digestible carbohydrates and fats, similar to the way modern grazing animals obtain all the nutrients they need from a diet of grasses. Evolution maximises energy efficiency and, there-fore, strips away unnecessary parts, like a longer intestine. The ability to digest plant fibres is a faculty that we humans lost because it was no longer needed. All that remains of that part of the digestive tract is our appendix.

Another evolutionary change from our primate cousins is that we grew significantly bigger brains over a relatively short period of time, brains that are in large part made up of sat-urated fats and a high concentration of a particular type of polyunsaturated fat—docosahexaenoic acid, or DHA, known to many of us as a key constituent of fish oil. Our brains are loaded with DHA. It's difficult to formulate a real-istic scenario in which non-marine sources of DHA would have been sufficient to drive our rapid brain development.

Dr. Jack Kruse, in his book *The Epi-Paleo Rx*, makes a strong argument that the incorporation of seafood into the diet as early humans migrated along coastal pathways was the most likely condition that allowed for rapid growth and development of the brain. Dr. Kruse is a brilliant neurosurgeon and knows more than most about the physiology of the human brain. He maintains that "seafood contains all of the ingredients necessary to build a brain".

These two evolutionary changes—the shortened intestinal tract and the bigger brain—suggest that our ancestral diet included, at the very least, nutrient-dense foods and a good source of DHA, neither of which can be provided by a strict plant-based diet. Of this I am fairly certain: Our ancestors did not lose any sleep worrying about the high fat content of their diets. They ate high-fat foods and animal protein for hundreds of thousands of years without any evidence of heart disease.

Spoiled for Choice: The Human 'Gorilla Biscuit'

To get a sense of the way misalignments in our diet can significantly affect our health, we can look at what happens to gorillas in captivity. In *The Paleo Manifesto*, John Durant tells the story of Mokolo, a western lowland gorilla living at the Cleveland Metroparks Zoo in America. Mokolo, like many other zoo gorillas, had a bad health profile while living in captivity: obesity, metabolic syndrome, high blood pressure, elevated cholesterol and triglycerides and an enlarged heart indicative of heart disease. In fact,

Mokolo's health profile resembled that of many of his adult male human cousins. Heart disease is the number one killer of both gorillas and humans. Mokolo also suffered from diarrhea and bizarre behaviours such as regurgitation and plucking out his hair. But Mokolo didn't drink or smoke or eat fatty foods or red meat or do any of the things that are supposedly associated with heart disease. In fact, he was a vegan whose diet consisted of 'gorilla biscuits' containing all the nutrients scientifically determined to be necessary for maintaining the health of gorillas in captivity (sort of like their version of the recommended daily allowance), along with a few plants and fruits.

Researchers wondered if Mokolo's diet was contributing to his health issues. As part of a project involving a few other American zoos, staff at the Cleveland Zoo decided to change Mokolo's diet, replacing the gorilla biscuits with plants that more closely resembled what gorillas in the wild eat. After about a week on the new diet, Mokolo (and the other gorillas involved in the project) stopped having diarrhea, stopped regurgitating their food and did much less hair-plucking. Even more importantly, Mokolo's blood pressure and triglycerides dropped and he lost up to 15% of his bodyweight, even though he consumed twice as many calories. *The health profiles for Mokolo and the other gorillas in the project changed within a week of returning to the diet their bodies were designed by evolution to eat.* (Recall that I, too, experienced a rapid turnaround in my symptoms after a little over a week of dietary change—although hair-plucking was never an issue!)

We in the Western world have our own version of the gorilla biscuit: the 'British Eatwell Plate', which is a version of its American cousin, 'The USDA Food Pyramid'. These dietary recommendations are what the professional dietary bodies in each of these two countries promote as the answer to the question, "What should we be eating for maximum health?" Let's examine what this human version of the gorilla biscuit looks like and then see if it creates any environmental misalignments that could be degrading our own health profiles.

The British Eatwell Plate, which has the endorsement of the Food Standards Agency (www.food.gov.uk), is a graphical image created to guide us in choosing the right proportions of five different food groups. These groups and their proportions, by volume, are:

1. Bread, rice, potatoes, pasta and other starchy foods (30%)

2. Fruit and vegetables (30%)

3. Meat, fish, eggs, beans and other non-dairy protein (15%)

4. Milk and dairy products (15%)

5. Foods and drinks high in fat and/or sugar (10%)

As you look at the Eatwell Plate recommendations and compare them to the hunter-gatherer diet from Paleolithic (Stone Age) times, you'll see a large percentage of foods on the Eatwell Plate that were never part of our ancestral diet: grains and cereals, beans and pulses, milk and dairy products of all kinds, processed and grain-fed meats, manufactured seed oils, sugars, and fruit and vegetables outside their short growing season or geographical area. In other words, the majority of what is on the plate wasn't part of our ancestral diet. Many of those foods, in fact, didn't even exist in our grandparents' time, much less in our ancestral cousins' time.

Our modern diet is truly a gorilla biscuit experiment of epic proportions—and it has epic consequences, as we shall see!

How did we get to this place?

From Evolution to Revolution: What Have We Done to Our Food Chain?

The transition from our ancestral hunter-gatherer diet to the Western diet of today was facilitated by two major historical events: the Agricultural Revolution and the Industrial Revolution. The first of these, the Agricultural Revolution, occurred between 7,000 and 10,000 years ago. Up until that time, most of the starchy foods that comprise 30% of the modern-day recommended diet didn't exist in the human diet. Grains, in particular, didn't feature highly, if at all. That includes the wheat, oats, rye, barley, rice and corn that have become a dominant portion of our diet. When our ancestors began to cultivate their own food, non-migratory civilisations developed and storage became possible for foods such as tubers, grains and flours, which could thus provide sustenance when other sources were scarce. The domestication of animals as livestock developed around that time as well, allowing dairy products to enter the diet.

The second major event, the Industrial Revolution, began in the mid to late 1800s and made the following possible:

- The mass production of crops through mechanised farming methods, and the application of pesticides, herbicides and chemical fertilisers;

- The creation of new varieties of crops through hybridisation and genetic modification;

- The mass production of animals and animal products through the use of grain-based feeds (sometimes fortified with hormones and antibiotics for rapid weight gain), as well as feedlot and battery cage practices;

- The industrial manufacturing of new food products that the human gut had never before been exposed to, such as seed oils, hydrogenated oils, refined or processed sugars (including high-fructose corn syrup), vegetable protein substitutes (such as soy), and artificial everything—sweeteners, flavourings, colourings and preservatives.

Even foods that were a stable part of the hunter-gatherer diet have been modified for our modern-day diet, sometimes beyond all recognition.

"Well, haven't we evolved to be able to consume this new diet?" you might ask. In terms of generations, if we estimate roughly 30 generations per 1,000 years, humans have been eating a hunter-gatherer diet for at least 200,000 years, or 6,000 generations. The Agricultural Revolution happened no more than 300 generations ago, and most of the changes following the Industrial Revolution have occurred over only the last three generations—many over the past three decades, or *a single lifetime*. If we were hoping that our bodies would have evolved to cope with these massive changes in our diet, here's a newsflash: There haven't been nearly enough years for that to happen!

Clearly, our diet today is not a match to the diet we evolved with through thousands of generations. Let's look more closely at those misalignments to see how our gorilla biscuit diet may be causing a physiological revolution that's manifesting as modern-day diseases. One way to do this is to look at the three major macronutrients—carbohydrates, fats and proteins—and the role each of them play in the make-up and function of our bodies.

A Carb-aholic Nightmare

Carbohydrates are the foods we think of as providing 'instant energy' and are found in high concentrations in starchy foods and sugars, in moderate concentrations in fruits and starchy vegetables—such as carrots and squash, and in low concentrations in most other vegetables. Carbohydrates are the hot-burning pine logs in my wood-burning-stove metaphor. More than 60% of the British Eatwell Plate consists of carbohydrates, when we combine the starchy foods with the fruits and vegetables and include the beans and sugars from other categories.

Carbohydrates, whatever their form, break down in the digestive system and are converted into the simple sugars glucose and fructose. Conventional wisdom tells us we need a steady stream of glucose available for energy, especially for the two biggest energy hogs in our bodies: the brain and the heart. Three square meals a day are recommended, with some snacks in between, to ensure we have a constant input of energy.

Our ancestors, though, did not have diets loaded with starches and sugars. Nor did they have food available round the clock, as we do. Besides fruits in season, the carbohydrate load of our Paleolithic cousins was comparatively very low. Evolution designed the human body to store some glucose in the form of glycogen in the liver and muscles, and to generate insulin to keep the level of glucose in the bloodstream within acceptable levels, because high levels of glucose are toxic to our tissues. A constant high level of carbohydrates in the diet is a misalignment, putting our blood sugar-regulating systems into overdrive and leaving our bodies swimming in insulin, a condition that signals the body to convert the excess glucose to fat and to store it for our survival (more about that later).

Life evolves in the direction of improved survival of the individual and the species. This is every bit as true for the plants we eat as it is for us humans. Let's take grains, for example. Grains are the seeds of grasses, and they need to stay on the stalk long enough to mature. How do they survive? They have to be able to resist all the critters that would munch them before they have a chance to mature and spread. One of the protective mechanisms of grains has been the development of proteins (such as glutens, phytates and lectins) that irritate the gut of animals that ingest them—including humans. Non-human animals learned over time not to eat grains because they made them sick. We didn't.

Many people are now aware of gluten as a source of digestive problems, which has spawned a whole industry around gluten-free foods. Coeliac disease is an extreme allergy to gluten (which is actually a whole family of proteins). Gluten sensitivity—a less severe form of gluten intolerance than coeliac disease—is much more widespread than originally thought, although it's not recognised by a large part of the medical establishment. Often, gluten sensitivity is difficult to diagnose because, unlike with Coeliac disease, the symptoms may appear outside of the gut in other areas of the body. Also, inflammation makes the gut lining more permeable—resulting in 'leaky gut', a condition which allows partially digested food particles and microbes to leak from the gut into the bloodstream, causing immune reactions.

Phytates and lectins have an irritating effect on the gut lining, and they also have the ability to bind to minerals, such as iron and magnesium, preventing their absorption. Because of this effect, phytates and lectins are sometimes referred to as 'antinutrients'—not only do they not giveth, they taketh away!

The grains we consume today are very different to those first cultivated 10,000 years ago. Most of our present-day grains are now hybridized beyond all resemblance to those our ancestors ate. Especially in the U.S., they've often been genetically modified as well. This is why many people who have sensitivities to other grains are able to tolerate spelt, which is a form of wheat closer to what was originally cultivated.

Genetically modified grains are now being exported to developing countries as livestock feed and seed for crops in order to increase yields. While GMO (genetically modified organisms) crops have, so far, been banned in Europe, they find their way into our food chain through animal feed and imported meats. Many small seed companies have been bought out or driven out of business by large companies, such as Monsanto and DuPont, and it has thus become more and more difficult for farmers in the U.S. and elsewhere to obtain seeds to grow non-GMO crops. In this way, a few very large companies have gained control over a significant portion of the global food chain.

Other foods besides grains contain phytates and lectins. Beans and pulses contain high levels of these proteins, with some of the highest concentrations found in soybeans. Many of our more recent ancestors developed techniques such as soaking, slow-cooking, and fermentation to break down these protein substances and render them more digestible. Slow-cooking lentils, for example, breaks down over 90% of the phytates they contain, and the same thing happens to soy during the Japanese practice of fermenting.

Then there are the sugars, which are getting a lot of press these days. Non-fruit sugars were not generally a part of the ancestral diet for most of our history. Though the cultivation of sugar cane dates back thousands of years (presses that could extract the juice more effectively were developed as far back as the 1300s), sugar was, for a long time, a precious and expensive commodity that didn't really find its way into any but the most wealthy households. That began to change in the late 1700s when the slave trade in the British and French colonies in the West Indies resulted in increased sugarcane production. In the mid 1800s, production increased even more when it became mechanised. By the 1900s, consumption of sugar was on the rise—and so was heart disease.

In the 1970s, a British scientist by the name of John Yudkin began to sound the alarm about the link between the high consumption of sugars and the rising incidence of cardiovascular disease. He was ignored and dismissed in favour of another theory—that saturated fat in our diet causes a rise in cholesterol which, in turn, leads to heart disease. Only now, 40 years later, are medical and dietary experts finally coming to realise that Yudkin may have been right after all.

Fructose is a sugar that is contained in fruits, and so would have been a part of the diet of many of our Paleolithic ancestors. Fructose is metabolised by the body in a completely different way to glucose. Once fructose is absorbed by the intestines it gets transported straight to the liver, where it's treated in a very similar way to alcohol: it's converted into fatty acid compounds call 'triglycerides', which are then usually stored as fat.

Fructose metabolism is a very handy evolutionary design, if you happen to be a mammal who lives in a region that undergoes significant seasonal changes in food availability. A high consumption of in-season fruits ensures the creation and storage of body fat that's then available for fuelling the body during winter, when other food sources are scarce. Think of those bears that fatten up on berries over the summer and then sleep it off in the winter. We may not hibernate in winter, but we've been designed to use up our fat stores during periods when food is less plentiful.

A product that has emerged out of our ability to manufacture foods is high fructose corn syrup (HFCS), which is derived, as its name suggests, from corn. It's about four times sweeter than table sugar. When high tariffs made sugar very expensive, and when an overproduction of corn drove its price down, the stage was set for replacing sugar with HFCS in thousands of products, from fizzy drinks to processed meats. With the low-fat craze creating a wave of fat-free or reduced-fat products, something had to be added to put some flavour back into those foods, and HFCS was the choice of many manufacturers.

HFCS is even added to savoury foods to improve their flavour and shelf life. As a result, our Western diet is filled with hidden sugars that are taxing not only our pancreas' ability to keep up the insulin production but also our liver's ability to convert all that fructose and to store the fats it produces.

Non-alcoholic fatty liver disease (NAFLD) has now surpassed the incidence of alcoholic liver disease and results in the same damaging effects. NAFLD is an adaptation to our environment. It is the body's way of doing its level best to keep up with a rate of sugar intake it was never designed to handle.

A Calorie Is a Calorie... Or Is It?

Another adaptation to our carb-laden diet is one that's becoming epidemic: obesity. Conventional wisdom has a lot to say about eating. For example, it says that "a calorie is a calorie" and that maintenance of a healthy weight is simply a matter of balancing "calories in and calories out". That means it doesn't matter what we eat, really, only that we keep track of the total calories we consume each day and balance that against an equal amount of calories burned through physical exercise. Heavens, we even have exercise machines that calculate calories burned and mobile phone apps to help us calculate and tally up the calories we consume throughout the day. How hard can it be to lose weight with that simple concept and all those tools? And if it's so simple, why are so many of us struggling with obesity? Conventional wisdom (and perhaps your healthcare provider) will attribute it to the two cardinal sins—gluttony and sloth—and tell you just to eat less and exercise more. Job done.

There was a time when I decided finally to lose those extra pounds—again—and so I started running daily while cutting back my calorie consumption through a low-fat diet, as conventional wisdom ordained. My weight did drop initially, but then it tapered off after only a couple of weeks. Even though I was running over two miles a day and consuming no more than 1200 calories a day, my weight plateaued. How was that even possible?

My metabolic rate *without* the running should have been burning all the calories I was eating. If losing weight is a matter of calories in minus calories out, then how come I wasn't losing any weight? Running over two miles a day every day was not sustainable, nor was the diet I was eating, so I gave up the running and returned to a more normal caloric intake. The weight flew back on, plus a little more. Again.

It Really Is Just My Hormones

Evolution designed us to manage our weight without dieting or counting calories or cross-fitting, and through times of feast and famine. Somehow, our ancestors had to manage without three meals a day through seasonal changes that controlled the availability of food sources, with no supermarket just down the block. Our survival as a species clearly suggests that evolution accounted for a highly variable food intake as we evolved.

Obesity is not a failing of will but a sign that something is broken in the body's system, that the internal regulator is not functioning as it should. Obesity is not a disease in itself but a symptom of underlying dysfunction. So, what is that control system that nature designed for us?

It is helpful first to understand that we have hybrid engines that run on two types of fuel, just like a hybrid car does. The hybrid car I used to drive ran on petrol power for acceleration and battery power for the rest of the time. The battery contained stored energy—using that as much as possible increased the efficiency of the engine. Our human hybrid engines run on glucose and a breakdown product of fats known as 'ketones'. Most of us are familiar with the concept of burning glucose in our cells to generate the energy needed to power life. But many of us have the misconception that when we 'burn fat' it's somehow converted to glucose. It is not. Glucose is a separate fuel. A car's hybrid engine and our hybrid engines function efficiently when they know which fuel to draw upon when, and how to build up and utilise stored energy.

How do our bodies know when to store fat and when to burn it? It manages this process by using a whole series of bossy hormones. Body fat, or adipose tissue, as it is more formally called, is more than just stored energy—it's living tissue. In 1994, Dr. Jeff Friedman at Rockefeller University discovered a previously unknown hormone called 'leptin' that is excreted from fat cells and circulates through the blood to the brain. A part of the brain known as the 'hypothalamus' functions as a kind of 'bean-counter' for fat cells. It does this by using leptin receptors to sense the amount of leptin in the bloodstream. More fat means more leptin and so the bean-counter knows how much fat is available. How cool is that? Leptin is also released after eating, to let the brain know that the body has adequate fuel.

Under normal functioning, when leptin levels are high, the brain will interpret that as meaning there's enough fuel in the system and will send signals to suppress the appetite, giving the command to "Stop eating!" It will also initiate the release of glucagon, giving the command to "Burn fat!" This is the body's response to a feast scenario.

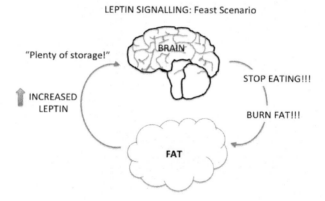

LEPTIN SIGNALLING: Feast Scenario

"Plenty of storage!"
BRAIN
STOP EATING!!!
INCREASED LEPTIN
BURN FAT!!!
FAT

Conversely, when leptin levels are low, the brain interprets that as not having enough reserve and orders the release of a hormone called 'ghrelin', which stimulates the appetite, giving the command "Eat!" It also stimulates the release of insulin, which gives the command to "Store fat!" This is the body's response to a famine scenario. If this situation continued for some time, as during a prolonged fast or starvation, the brain would also downregulate metabolism and shut of all non-vital functions (such as fertility) to conserve energy.

LEPTIN SIGNALLING: Famine Scenario

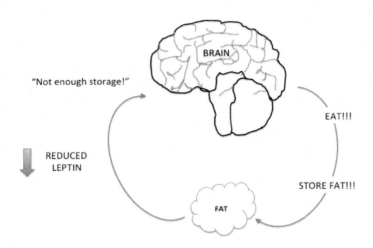

What happens as a result of our carb-laden diet is that our bodies are swimming in insulin. Insulin turns off fat burning and initiates fat storage, which puts more leptin into circulation. Over time, in the presence of continuously high leptin levels, the leptin receptors become insensitive to the signal, a condition known as leptin resistance. Now the leptin bean-counter can't tell that there are adequate fat stores. It thinks the body's is in a famine scenario and continues to give out appetite stimulation and fat storage signals. It also downregulates the metabolism because it thinks starvation is imminent.

At this point, the system is broken and we have the metabolic paradox of a person who is obese and starving at the same time. They're hungry all the time, driven by cravings for high-energy carbohydrates, and also tired much of the time, due to a low metabolic rate. Urging that person to cut their caloric intake and exercise only raises their body's demand for energy and increases the starvation signal their body is already receiving. A crash diet can force them to lose weight, although often it's lean weight that's lost instead of fat weight, because the body breaks down muscle protein to convert it into glucose in its attempts to prevent starvation. When the crash diet is over, though, the body quickly compensates by replacing the fat plus a little extra as a buffer.

Obesity isn't due to gluttony or sloth. It isn't happening from a weakness of will. The system is broken and needs resetting. Fortunately, this is possible to do.

On his website, Dr. Kruse lays out a protocol he calls the Leptin Prescription which gives steps for regaining leptin sensitivity while shedding excess weight. It's a high-protein, low-carbohydrate diet based on what is basically an ancestral template. Meals are timed in such a way that they override the broken signalling and retrain the brain. If you're someone who's struggling to shed abdominal fat and has tried many things without lasting success, what I want to say to you is that, first, it's not all your fault and, second, there's a way to fix it. I've used Dr. Kruse's leptin reset protocol myself and coached my clients through it, with great success.

Not All Fats Are Equal (or Evil)

In spite of the fact that humans have consumed high levels of fat over at least hundreds of thousands of years; that they make up a large portion of the human body, including our cell membranes, brain, and nervous system; that they form the backbone of all of our hormones; and that they are necessary for the absorption of essential vitamins and nutrients, they have been given a pretty bad rap for several decades. Conventional wisdom says that if we eat fat, we get fat. Everyone knows that fat contains more calories per unit weight than carbohydrates or proteins. Everyone knows fat clogs our arteries. That's what conventional wisdom (fuelled by faulty science) says. That's not the real story, however.

I remember going to the cinema in America in the 1960s and the delicious way popcorn used to taste and smell— different from what it's like today. The reason is that it used to be popped in coconut oil, because coconut oil was cheap and plentiful and didn't burn easily. Then coconut oil disappeared from our Western diet, practically overnight, along with butter and lard, only to be replaced by margarine, vegetable oil, and shortening (all hydrogenated oils).

Full-fat dairy products and fatty cuts of meat were replaced by skimmed milk and skinless chicken. 'Fat-Free' became the name of the game.

It seems that a researcher at the University of Minnesota by the name of Ancel Keys has a lot to answer for. He had a theory about fats that competed with Britain's John Yudkin's theory (about the high consumption of sugars and the rising incidence of cardiovascular disease). Keys set out to prove that the saturated fats in our diet were the real culprits in the rise of coronary heart disease. His theory, the Diet-Heart Hypothesis, states that a high intake of saturated fats raises blood cholesterol levels, which, in turn, causes heart disease. He set out to prove his theory by analysing data about the diets and incidence of heart disease in 22 countries. His 'Six Countries Analysis' graph depicts a nearly perfect curve showing the rate of heart disease rising as fat intake increased.

As Denise Minger details in her book *Death by Food Pyramid*, there were some significant flaws in his study and conclusions. First of all, the data from 22 countries were available, but Keys only presented the results of six. When data from the remaining countries are added to the Six Countries Analysis graph, one is hard pressed to find any relationship between heart disease and fat intake, let alone the same strong correlation as with his cherry-picked six-country data. Secondly, his results for the six countries of his graph only showed a *correlation* between fat consumption and heart disease. 'Correlation' is not the same as 'causation', though it's often interpreted and reported as such. Just because two things trend in the same direction does not mean that one causes the other, or even that they are related.

Researchers ridiculed Keys' methods and results. Still, he was able to sell his ideas to the U.S. Government at a time when America's silos were sitting full from overproduction. Corn oil and soybean oil had already been developed for industrial purposes, such as in paints, but they didn't originally have any dietary use. Keys' study, implying that removing saturated fats from the diet would prevent heart disease, conveniently paved the way for replacing saturated fats with industrial oils. Perhaps that's why the flaws in Keys' conclusions, pointed out by many other academics at the time, were overlooked. It probably also helped that the American diet was about to be redesigned by the U.S. Department of Agriculture (USDA). Not the American Medical Association, as one might expect for an issue so central to our health, but the USDA, whose job is to protect the American food industry.

The Diet-Heart Hypothesis has been tested in multiple studies since Keys first presented his analysis. Even though most reviewers of his theory now conclude that diets that are high in fat do not result in a greater incidence of heart disease; even though it is known that Keys' studies were flawed, the old message persists.

Fuelling the Inflammatory Flames

"What is the problem with manufactured oils and fats?" you might wonder. After all, don't they reduce cholesterol? This is a case of 'you are what you eat'. The fats we consume are not only burned as fuel for energy in our hybrid engines, they're incorporated into biological structures, such as our cell membranes, the myelin sheaths that protect our nerves, and our hormones. What we eat, we become. Manufactured oils are not nature's oils, and they cause problems for us when our bodies are loaded with them. Let's see why.

Two very important types of polyunsaturated fatty acids (PUFAs) are tied to immune function: omega-6 fatty acids (O6) and omega-3 fatty acids (O3). Omega-6 fatty acids are pro-inflammatory, while omega-3 fatty acids are anti-inflammatory. Both are needed by the body—we need to fire up the immune system to fight off infections, for example, and we need to be able to cool the inflammation when the infection is resolved.

Evidence suggests that we evolved around a diet very evenly balanced between the two PUFAs—a balance of O6:O3 that's roughly 1:1. Seed oils (such as corn oil, soybean oil or 'vegetable oil') are high in pro-inflammatory O6 fatty acids. By replacing saturated fats with these seed oils in our Western diet we have elevated our O6:O3 ratios, with estimates ranging from 10:1 to 28:1. The result is systemic inflammation, which is seriously bad news, as it not only contributes to heart disease, but also to cancer, obesity, dementias, infertility, and so much more.

Further, the hydrogenated versions of the industrial seed oils, called 'trans fats' (margarine is an example), have been shown to be directly linked to increased incidence of heart disease. The 'cure' has become the cause.

Not only is it true that we are what we eat, we are what *they* eat as well. One of the big changes in animal husbandry has involved a change in the animals' diets in order to produce bigger, fatter animals faster. Take cows, for example. Grazing in pastures is the natural way cows feed, but it's not as fast or efficient as cattle producers wanted it to be. In ranching, the weight of the animals and speed of production matter to the financial bottom line. Feedlots allow more cattle to be raised in a smaller space. By feeding cows corn and soybeans instead of allowing them to graze in pastures, they grow fatter faster. They do this because the unnatural feed they're given destroys the rumen, the magical part of their digestive systems that allows cows to turn grass into the nutrients they need. This causes inflammation and infections, because of the absorption of bacteria through the damaged rumen, and that requires treatment by antibiotics. This is not dissimilar to how eating a gorilla biscuit diet creates havoc in the human gut, causing systemic inflammation, leaky gut and obesity. We, too, get fatter faster.

The O3 oils normally produced by bacteria in a cow's rumen are replaced by O6 oils from the corn in their feed. The impact on us when we consume corn-fed beef is that we consume those higher levels of O6. Since we are what we eat *and* what they eat, this makes the already high O6:O3 ratio even worse. The same thing happens when we eat battery cage chickens and their eggs or any other feedlot animal that's being fed an unnatural diet—their version of the gorilla biscuit.

Evolution's High-Octane Fuel

The human body does not produce all the fats it needs in the same way that grazing animals or even our gorilla cousins do. Fat is an essential food and we evolved by consuming it in our diet—lots of it. When fat is broken down to use as fuel, ketones are formed. 'Ketosis' is a condition of elevated levels of ketones in the body as the body burns fat for fuel. We commonly go in and out of ketosis, especially at night, when most fat-burning occurs. Ketosis is a natural function of the body and is not the same thing as 'ketoacidosis', a condition that most commonly occurs with diabetes and that is dangerous. Conventional wisdom says that our brains need constant glucose to function, but it turns out that our brains and hearts work more efficiently on ketones than glucose.

Imagine if you were in charge of evolution and had to design the human body in such a way that it could run primarily on stored fats during lean times. Which two organs are so crucial to life they're at the top of the list of ketone burners? The heart and the brain, of course. The ability of the brain to function effectively using ketones is why there have been cases of people suffering from Alzheimer's Disease doing better when coconut oil, which breaks down readily into ketones, is added to their diet. With Alzheimer's, glucose metabolism in the brain is disrupted, accelerating tissue death. For this reason, Alzheimer's is sometimes referred to as 'Type 3 diabetes'. Ketones, like those from coconut oil, help to bypass this problem because they metabolise differently in the mitochondria than glucose does.

Fats are nature's high-octane fuel. Evolution designed our bodies to use them, not just as an occasional back up when carbs are scarce, but as a preferred fuel for our most critical organs. Lady Evolution would bang her head on the desk about our 'low fat' craze!

Cholesterol: A Red Herring

Thanks to Keys' Diet-Heart Hypothesis, cholesterol has been cast as an evil force to be banished from our diet and our bodies at all costs. Thus, it has become the target of many dietary and pharmaceutical interventions intended to reduce the incidence of heart disease. Perhaps the best known of the pharmaceutical interventions are a family of cholesterol-lowering medications called 'statins'. Studies show that statins don't affect mortality one whit. Meanwhile, side effects from taking statins abound, although drug manufacturers play down their incidence and severity.

In *The Statin Damage Crisis*, Duane Graveline describes how statins work to reduce cholesterol. They are indeed very effective at blocking the production of cholesterol, but they unfortunately also block the formation of other essential substances that the body needs, resulting in collateral damage.

Statins are a multi-billion-dollar business. If heart disease can continue to be blamed on high cholesterol and if the recommended 'healthy' level of cholesterol continues to be lowered, as it has over the past decade, then statins will continue to be a gravy train for the pharmaceutical industry for many years to come.

Here's the problem: Our bodies cannot function without adequate levels of cholesterol. It's so critical to our survival that evolution designed our bodies with the capacity to *make our own* cholesterol. When cholesterol levels drop, the liver makes more of it. Cholesterol is the backbone of all our hormones, including vitamin D (which is actually a hormone, not a vitamin). It is also a key component of cell membranes, the brain and the myelin sheaths surrounding nerves. The effects of too little cholesterol are far more dangerous than the effects of too much of it.

The link between cholesterol and heart disease was made through the discovery that cholesterol is a component of the fatty plaques that line the arteries in cases of heart disease. Cholesterol has been portrayed as dangerous blobs of fat floating through the bloodstream and sticking to the walls of blood vessels, like grease in your water pipes, eventually completely blocking the arteries and causing heart attacks. But that is not an accurate picture.

It is now known that inflammatory processes cause injury to the blood vessel walls and cholesterol may be the body's way to try to patch those injuries. The concern about cholesterol is not whether it's the high-density (HDL) "good cholesterol" or the low-density (LDL) "bad cholesterol" (both are actually needed by the body), but whether or not the cholesterol is oxidised. Oxidation causes the formation of "free radicals" that can damage tissue, like what happens when metal gets rusty.

LDL cholesterol comes in different shapes and sizes, from small, dense particles to large, fluffy ones. The small, dense particles are particularly susceptible to oxidation while the large fluffy ones are not. Most doctors don't test for cholesterol size when doing lipid profiles (you can get those tests done on your own), yet they do test for triglycerides, which can indicate the presence of smaller cholesterol particles, since the levels of the two are correlated. So you can look at your own blood tests and see how you're doing by whether or not your triglyceride level is high. What you want are more of the larger, fluffier cholesterol particles and fewer of the small, dense ones.

So, what causes an increase in the small, dense type of cholesterol? It's not fat in the diet, as you might think. It is high levels of carbohydrates, especially fructose. Drop the level of starchy carbs and sugars in your diet, and you will see those small, dense cholesterol levels go down, along with your triglycerides.

Saturated fats, such as coconut oil and animal fats, are not an evolutionary mismatch. But industrial seed oils are. We're not designed to *avoid* cholesterol; we're designed to *manufacture* it. Cholesterol is not the issue, and statins or other interventions (such as 'cholesterol-lowering' butter replacement spreads), are not the solution. Heart disease is the body's adaptation to a carb-rich, inflammatory diet we were not designed to consume.

A Word About Proteins

Protein can be used as a back up fuel when amino acids, the building blocks of protein, are converted into glucose. However, a more essential use of proteins is that the amino acids they contain become the building blocks for the thousands of proteins our bodies use. DNA is basically a blueprint for building proteins, and proteins are critical to all levels of functioning. They make up a large portion of most tissues. They allow communication within and between cells. They form the enzymes that initiate biochemical reactions, the neurotransmitters that allow our nerves to transmit signals, the hormones that allow the brain to control and coordinate various processes throughout the body, and the biological 'wires' that allow energy transmissions to occur.

Although our bodies are capable of converting some amino acids into others, there are some essential amino acids that the body cannot manufacture. Therefore, they have to be obtained through the diet. Not only does our modern diet have to contain a wide enough source of proteins to provide those essential amino acids, but the ancestral diet had to have contained those sources, too. If evolution didn't design the means to make it, it stands to reason there was a sufficient source of it in the environment that we could ingest. This means that we not only require enough protein in our diet, but enough of the right kinds, as well.

Today's vegans are challenged to find non-animal protein sources that provide adequate amounts of the whole spectrum of essential amino acids, even with access to today's supermarkets and the unnatural availability and wide range of foods they offer. Imagine how tough it would have been for our early ancestors trying to forage for those vegan protein sources year-round within a limited geographical area!

A meat-based or meat- and plant-based diet will easily provide a year-round source of the essential amino acids the body doesn't produce. It will also provide essential fatty acids, vitamins, minerals and other micronutrients, especially when more of the whole animal is eaten, nose to tail, as our ancestors did.

Realign With Your Design

So, going back to our modern day gorilla biscuit diet, here are the foods that we commonly eat today that were not part of our ancestral diet: all grains and grain flours, legumes and pulses, seed oils, milk and dairy products, processed foods of any kind, refined sugars, fruits out of season and locality, grain-fed meat and poultry, and artificial any-thing. You now know why they cause havoc for a large per-centage of us today. Just because we *can* manufacture and consume a gorilla-biscuit diet doesn't mean that we *should*.

Biology always wins. It doesn't care about your dietary pref-erences or whether or not you're on holiday. It doesn't care if preparing healthy foods is inconvenient or that you have religious or ethical reasons to avoid certain foods. It doesn't care if you're thrilled about being able to purchase tropical fruits in high latitudes year-round or if salted caramel ice cream is just too good to resist. We ignore our evolutionary design at our peril.

You might be sucking air at this point, worried about seeing some of your favourite foods in the categories I listed above and wondering what's left for you to eat that is enjoyable and tasty. Here's what's left: grass-fed, free range, pastured meats, poultry, and eggs; vegetables of all sizes, shapes, and colours; local fruits in season; tubers, as tolerated, espe-cially sweet potatoes when in season; seeds and nuts; fish of every kind; the whole range of herbs and spices; full-fat dairy, for those who can tolerate it; and, best of all, healthy fats such as coconut oil, butter, full-fat cream, duck fat, lard, olive oil, nut oils, avocados—all those fabulously lovely fats that used to be part of our diet until flawed science and gov-ernment policy determined that they were detrimental to our health and gave us trans fats instead.

How do we go about correcting the evolutionary mis-matches? We simply remove from our diet what didn't used to be part of it for hundreds of thousands of years and put back what was part of it. This means eating local foods in season and eating whole foods in their natural states. If we live in latitudes closer to the poles, where sun exposure is limited much of the year, we add even more seafood to our diets. We invest in the additional cost of buying high-quality organic foods, because we either pay now (for quality) or we pay dearly later on (for expensive medical care).

In the long run, it pays to align our diets with how evolution designed us to function. But don't just take my word for it. Be an evolutionary explorer. Have a look at your Get Started Questionnaire (evolutionaryreboot.com/get-started -questionnaire) to identify where the misalignments are in your own diet, then do your own gorilla-biscuit-free experiments. Capture data as you go. Record the changes as you try different things and let your experience teach you.

P.S. Knives and forks are still allowed!

CHAPTER FOUR

The Light of Your Life

"I think you might dispense with half your doctors if you would only consult Dr. Sun more." **HENRY WARD BEECHER**

Sleep is a funny thing. On a weekend morning a good lie-in feels like such a luxury. At other times, it seems an inconvenience and a waste of valuable time that could be better spent doing other things. Being able to manage on just a few hours of sleep has become, for many, a sort of badge of honour. Mother Nature should surely have designed a better system, one that allows us to survive on cat-naps during the week and then load up on sleep during weekends—sleeping the same number of hours overall, but redistributed. Many of us do, in fact, live as if we were designed that way, and we seem to get away with it, at least for a while. I know I certainly did during my decades in the research world with its 60-hour+ weeks and constant deadlines.

When I ask people, "How much sleep is enough?" I get answers ranging from the standard "eight hours a night" to "however many hours so that you don't feel tired". Some sleep experts suggest that some of us are 'night owls' while others of us are 'morning people', and we need to adjust our sleep habits according to those needs. According to *The Great British Bedtime Report* (2013), more than one-third of us slept for only five to six hours per night, a 7% increase over the previous 3 years. An average night's sleep 100 years ago, in Western countries, was 8.5 hours.

A recent article in a London newspaper suggested that we start our workdays too early and that children shouldn't even begin classes until ten or eleven in the morning. That recommendation misses a very important piece of the picture that could explain why many adults and children aren't running on all cylinders until mid- to late-morning (you'll know that piece by the end of this chapter). This is yet another example of trying to put a plaster on a problem rather than treating the underlying issue.

A common complaint I hear, and one I experienced for years, is an inability to fall asleep or stay asleep, even when there's time available for sleeping. It's that feeling of being 'tired and wired'—in bed, but lying there for a long time before dropping off, then waking up after only 2 or 3 hours and going through the whole thing again. And then dragging yourself out of bed in the morning, feeling like death warmed up, waiting impatiently for that double espresso to slap you into wakefulness. If that's you, chances are your body clocks are broken. That's not a good sign.

Circadian Signals and How Our Bodies Tell Time

So many different processes occur within our bodies that one might wonder how all those activities are coordinated. Many of us are familiar with the term 'circadian rhythms', which refers to the way certain body functions operate on a 24-hour pattern. But who or what is conducting this grand orchestra of organs, tissues and cells so that we end up with a harmonious symphony rather than a disjointed cacophony?

Evolution has enabled us to utilise our environment to tell time. We evolved within cycles of light and darkness, and our bodies have built-in clocks that help coordination happen. Coordinating around light requires our bodies to be sensitive to light, and so evolution gave us a set of photovoltaic cells and solar panels that are built into our eyes, brain and skin.

Evolution gave us both photovoltaic cells and solar panels long before we invented the technology. Photovoltaic cells operate like light sensors in streetlights that sense when evening comes and automatically turn on the light. Solar panels absorb sunlight and convert it into energy.

Our bodies are powered and regulated by sunlight, every bit as much as the plants around us. The human brain developed a Timex long before we became dependent on the one on our wrist. Circadian signalling from our internal clocks controls things like metabolism, hormone levels, temperature, sleep, tissue regeneration and repair, brain physiology, learning, memory and cognition, immune system restoration and even gene expression. In other words, if our body clocks are broken, we are in deep doo-doo. And here's the thing: The lion's share of restoration and repair happens when we sleep.

When I was in nursing school, ages ago, I learned that the pineal gland contains light sensors that were, at that time, thought be a relict of evolution, something we don't really need that's been passed along through millions of years since human life's early beginnings. But form follows function, and evolution always streamlines to remove what is obsolete. In other words, if it's in the body, it has a purpose. We now know that the pineal gland receives light signals through the pupils of the eyes, transmitting those signals directly to the brain, which uses them to coordinate bodily processes. The master controller in our brain is powered by light, but not just any light. It turns out that that our light sensors are most sensitive to wavelengths in a particular part of the light spectrum: the wavelengths that range from ultraviolet to visible blue light.

We are designed to sense blue light at sunrise, to be awake during the light part of the 24-hour day, to sense the change in the frequency of blue light at sunset, and to sleep in darkness. Our early ancestors spent their lives outdoors, continually exposed to those natural light cycles. I suspect they had little difficulty sleeping!

I once spent 3 months hiking the Appalachian Trail, sleeping in shelters or in a tent the whole time. I can tell you that it wasn't long before my body was in tune with light and darkness. Sleep came like clockwork within a few hours of sunset and my body was wide-awake at first light, without the use of an alarm. Blue light tells our bodies to wake up, to raise our metabolic rate, to go find food, to get moving.

Here's the problem: With the Industrial Revolution came Thomas Edison and the development of artificial light. We now have the capability to extend 'day' as long as we wish. Worse yet, the Technological Revolution we're in now has brought us ever more sophisticated forms of lighting and a wide variety of backlit devices, such as computers, tablets and smart phones. Our lights are brighter and more intense than Edison's original light bulbs, and that brightness can be attributed to one thing: a high concentration of blue light.

Our brain cannot tell the difference between blue light from the sun and blue light from an iPhone. The brain communicates in the language of frequencies and wavelengths. This means that when we use our computers at night, when we light up our homes, when we watch television, when we read our iBooks or check our phones for messages, our brains get the message that it's daytime—time to wake up, to jack up metabolism, go find food, get moving. We're getting a morning message late at night.

Blue light shreds sleep, full stop. It destroys melatonin production and therefore disrupts the entire hormonal cascade that happens at night to put us to sleep and to repair and restore our bodies. Blue light toxicity is disrupting circadian signalling and destroying our biological clocks. In our blue-lit cities, the level of light pollution is so bad it even disrupts the feeding and breeding behaviour of birds in the area. Is there any wonder the Western world is chronically sleep-deprived and chronically sick?

Remember that I said earlier that diet is not the most important thing to get right in order to regain your health? A good diet will not fix a bad environment, and artificial blue light creates one of the worst environments for us. We need only look at what really happens when we sleep to fully comprehend the implications for our health of not allowing and supporting our natural circadian rhythms.

Human Hibernation

Many animals hibernate through part of the year. Evolution designed them to build up and store energy in the form of fat over the long light cycles of summer, and then to live off of those fat stores through the short days of winter. During hibernation their systems are restored and repaired, and they emerge from their hibernation hungry, but with enough energy to search for food.

Why don't we humans hibernate? Well, actually, we do. We just do it in short bursts, at night. We may think that our bodies pretty much shut down for the night while we sleep, but a lot goes on. What goes on while we sleep is so critical to our health that sleep deprivation can lead to illness, obesity, cognitive decline, psychosis or even death. Perhaps sleep is not a waste of time after all.

A whole cascade of hormone-driven processes occurs through the night. Each step of that cascade appears to be dependent on the previous steps. If we don't start out right at the beginning, the whole cascade falls apart.

The sleep cascade starts with darkness—specifically, an absence of blue light. After 3 to 4 hours of darkness, and when the levels of a hormone called 'cortisol' (the stress hormone) drop, the pineal gland begins to secrete a hormone called 'melatonin', which many of us know as the 'sleep hormone', because it makes us drowsy, helps us fall asleep and helps us stay asleep. Melatonin secretion generally peaks between midnight and 2 am, so if you stay up late and don't get the requisite period of darkness, you miss the melatonin window and the cascade of restoration is disrupted.

Melatonin also opens up a gate in the brain that allows leptin into the hypothalamus. Leptin begins to be released from our fat cells early in the sleep cycle and continues through the night. The hypothalamus is the 'bean counter' of fat cells that I spoke about in the last chapter. It begins to do its magic at this stage, determining how much fat we have and if there's any excess to burn off.

After the release of melatonin, the pituitary gland releases the hormone 'prolactin', which, in turn, stimulates a process called 'myelinogenesis'. Myelin is the protective sheath surrounding all the nerves in our body, kind of like the insulation around an electrical cable. We need to be able to make myelin so we can repair damaged nerves, and in order to form new neural networks for memory storage.

We receive a lot of information and sensory input through-out the day. Our brains sift through all of that information, snipping out the bits that are not important and building new networks to capture and retain the important stuff. Myelinogenesis allows us to learn and remember. This process of myelinogenesis is also why babies and toddlers need so many more hours of sleep than adults—they are born with incompletely formed brains and need to build their brains during sleep.

Later in the sleep cycle, the pituitary gland releases 'growth hormone', which is responsible for protein turnover and immune system repair. The proteins in the body need to be replaced, either because they become damaged through use or injury or because they've simply reached their 'sell by' date. Growth hormone allows new proteins to be formed. Without it, the body has to recycle old and damaged ones. Our immune system also needs continuous replenishing. It's no coincidence that during times of sleep deprivation people are much more susceptible to illness. It's because the immune system has been weakened.

During the last couple of hours of sleep (in an 8-hour cycle) the pituitary gland tells the thyroid gland to increase metabolism, causing the hypothalamus to give the signal to burn off excess fat as pure heat, thus increasing body temperature. This is the part of the night when you might feel like ripping off the covers. We don't actually burn fat when we're on that CrossFit machine—we burn during sleep, *mainly during the last part of the night*. This is why sleep deprivation and short nights of sleep promote obesity!

The hormone cortisol, which is secreted by the adrenal glands, is supposed to be at its lowest at night as darkness descends. It then gradually rises through the night until morning, when it's at its peak. A drop in the cortisol level at day's end allows the body to become drowsy, and a spike of cortisol in the morning signals the body to wake up. It also stimulates the release of yet another hormone, 'ghrelin', which stimulates the appetite. Getting food was not so easy for our Paleolithic ancestors—not like walking to the refrigerator or driving to the local convenience store. So evolution built in a way to make sure humans would go to the effort of hunting game or gathering whatever edible plants were available: hunger. Hunger is intended to rise in the morning, and is an important part of the circadian pattern.

Here's a graphic representation of the sleep cycle and its effects on the body:

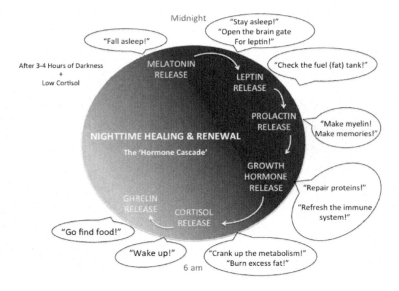

It takes between 7 and 9 hours to complete the full cycle. Any fewer hours and something in the process is short-changed or missed altogether. People not running on all cylinders until 10 or 11 in the morning may be doing so because of exposure to blue light from their computers and tablets the night before, which messed up the cascading sleep cycle.

You might be thinking, "Well I don't have a weight problem, so I can get away with shaving off those last couple of hours of sleep." You might want to think again, because of how memory and learning are affected by how long and how well we sleep.

"To Sleep, Perchance to Dream"

Dr. Robert O. Becker was an orthopaedic surgeon and a brilliant researcher who pioneered our understanding of the bioelectric properties of the body. In his book *The Body Electric* he describes his experiments aimed at understanding how the body heals and how tissues regenerate. I will say more about this in the next chapter, but what is pertinent here is what he discovered about electrical currents in the brain and their relationship to sleep.

Many of his experiments were conducted on salamanders and were aimed at detecting the natural electrical currents in their bodies that controlled certain physiological processes, including consciousness. He later extended those experiments to the human brain. What he discovered was that when we're awake electrical currents flow from the back of the brain to the front, but during sleep that direction reverses and electrical currents flow from the front to the back of the brain.

Through subsequent research by Dr. Olena Bukalo at the National Institutes of Health in America, it was discovered that when the electrical current changes direction during sleep it strips away unnecessary information and resets the brain so that it's ready to record new memories. Evolution has worked out a way for us to sift through all the information we're exposed to every day and retain only what's important. Out with the old, in with the new!

The brain goes through several of these cycles of forward and reverse currents each night, and different levels of sleep occur during these cycles. We have a different type of brainwave for every level of sleep, each with its own electrical signature, which is how researchers have been able to map out what the brain is up to at night and what 'normal' sleep looks like. Beta waves occur when we are fully awake. Alpha waves occur when we're still conscious, but our eyes are closed and we're becoming relaxed and drowsy. Alpha waves are also generated when we become relaxed during activities like meditation or listening to music, which is why engaging in these kinds of activities in the evening helps us fall asleep.

The first stage of sleep is a light sleep associated with theta waves. This is when the brain's electrical current reverses direction. We are now unconscious.

Next, we drop into the deep sleep associated with delta waves. As the cycle progresses, there's a brief return to light sleep, at which point the current changes direction again and we go into a phase known as 'rapid eye movement' (REM) sleep. This is the dreaming phase, a time when the brain is also actively involved in building memory and imprinting learning. In REM sleep, we're very close to the conscious state, and we might even spontaneously wake up for a brief time before dropping into the next cycle, especially in the early morning hours. The cycle begins anew when the brain goes back into a theta-wave state and the electrical current in the brain reverses again.

The following is a schematic that shows what a typical healthy pattern of sleep cycles might look like:

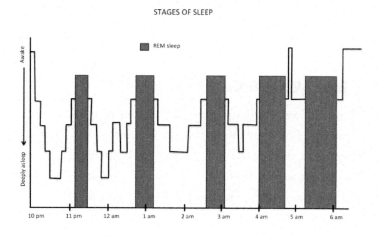

STAGES OF SLEEP

After Dement, W., *The Stanford Sleep Book*

As the night progresses, the cycles get shorter, sleep gets shallower, and REM cycles get longer. In a typical 8-hour night, we might go through this cycle 5 or 6 times, *with the last two hours of sleep dominated by REM sleep, the stage when memory and learning are built.* It appears that evolution designed these cycles into our sleep because building neural networks and storing memory requires repeatedly imprinting the memories to make them stick. It's similar to what we do when we repeatedly go over our times tables in order to memorise them. Our brain does that for us as we sleep, to help us embed our memories. Embedding starts about an hour into sleep, continues through the night and reaches its most intense level in the last hours of sleep. People suffering from sleep disturbances often report foggy thinking and poor memory. That's no surprise—if you cut your nights short, you also diminish your ability to learn and remember.

Our Built-In Solar Panels

So far, we've discussed sunlight's function in circadian timing. But what about its other functions? We know that sunlight is critical to plants. They have their own built-in solar panels in the form of leaves. Within those leaves is a sun-catching compound known as 'chlorophyll', the substance that gives plants their green colour. Energy from captured sunlight powers all the processes plants need in order to grow. Some of that energy gets stored in the plant's structure and is passed on to the animals that eat the plants.

Evolution has also equipped us humans with solar panels and sun-catching compounds. Our in-built solar panels are called 'skin' and our sun-catching compound is called 'haemoglobin' (the iron-rich substance in our red blood cells that gives our blood its red colour). I never learned this in nursing school or in any of my biology courses!

If evolution gave us these solar panels and sun-catching compounds, it stands to reason that we're meant to be getting lots of exposure to the sun, just as our early ancestors did. In fact, both chlorophyll and haemoglobin are designed to capture *all* wavelengths of ultraviolet light (UV)—even those we've labelled as 'dangerous'. We wouldn't think of covering our garden to hide it from sun exposure, but we don't think twice about hiding ourselves from sunlight. In fact, conventional wisdom has convinced us that exposure to sun is so dangerous we must slather on sunscreen at the first sign of the sun peeking out of the clouds, lest we burn or get skin cancer.

Let's look at this assumption for a moment through an evolutionary lens. Evolution gave us the equipment to catch the sun. Paleolithic humans were continuously exposed to the sun without developing skin cancer (which is also true for indigenous populations today). But, people in the Western world need to hide from the sun because exposure to it risks death. There is something very wrong with that perspective, which is out of alignment with how we evolved. Could this be affecting our health?

There is a complex story about what happens to the light our bodies capture. For now, I will use one process to illustrate what happens when we block ourselves from the sun.

Vitamin D is actually not a vitamin at all, but a mislabelled hormone crucial to many processes in our body. It's so critical, in fact, that every tissue in our body has vitamin D receptors. That means that every tissue in our body uses vitamin D to function. Because vitamin D is so critical, evolution has built in a way for our body to produce its own supply—by using sunlight absorbed through the skin. But not just any sunlight. This process requires UV light.

In spite of conventional wisdom about the evils of sunlight exposure—ideas that are deeply engrained in the dermatological community—there are a couple of confounding facts that contradict that 'wisdom'. One is that the incidence of skin cancer is higher at latitudes closer to the poles and drops nearer the equator where the sun is more intense. The other is that melanoma is now more common in people who use sunscreen. Hmm. Yet conventional wisdom carries on down that same path without examining these contradictions.

Looking through the evolutionary lens, we see that we weren't designed to get our vitamin D through supplements or fortified milk. Instead, we were designed to make our own. Those of us whose ancestors migrated to more northern latitudes, where sunlight is less intense, evolved to have lighter skin in order to capture *more* sunlight, not less! Our ancestors had to make the best of whatever light was available to them, for as much of the year as they could.

When the sun's energy gets more intense, like during the summer, our skin manufactures melanin, giving it a tan colour to block some of the more intense rays, allowing us to spend even more time in the sun and preventing us from burning. That's the way our bodies are designed by evolution to work in the presence of sunlight.

Without adequate vitamin D, we get sick. One of the more well known diseases caused by a vitamin D deficiency is rickets, a condition affecting the bones. What many people don't know is that vitamin D deficiency also contributes to heart disease, high blood pressure, obesity, arthritis, seizure disorders, mental illness, muscle weakness, immune deficiency and a wide variety of cancers. Since vitamin D receptors are in every tissue of our body, a deficiency affects a wide range of functions.

Skin cancer does affect us today—that is a fact, but it appears to be a recent development in human history. The sun hasn't changed. So, clearly, something we're doing has. Let's find the mismatch.

There's a chicken-and-egg situation with vitamin D and sunlight. We need sunlight to make vitamin D, but we also need vitamin D to protect our skin from some of the more damaging types of UV light. If things are working as they should, our body's natural protection system prevents the need for sunscreen. But vitamin D has to go through a whole series of steps to get to that active, skin-protecting form, and each step requires magnesium and water. Our modern diet is grossly lacking in magnesium, so much so that an estimated three-quarters of people in the Western world are deficient. The use of modern agricultural techniques and the heavy application of pesticides has stripped our soils of their natural levels of magnesium, resulting in far lower concentrations in the foods we eat than what was present just 50 years ago. To make matters worse, our modern carbohydrate-loaded diet and lifestyle keep us continuously dehydrated. Finally, a high ratio of omega-6 to omega-3 fatty acids (O6:O3) in our bodies leaves our skin more susceptible to cancer from UV exposure.

We can block the sun to try to prevent cancers, causing all sorts of other problems, or we can fix the mismatch and let our bodies work as they were designed to. Returning our diets to a Paleolithic template can restore our magnesium levels and bring our O6:O3 levels back into balance, particularly if a high level of seafood is incorporated into the diet.

There is an argument for using supplemental vitamin D and magnesium in the short term, to give the body time for the change in diet to take effect and for natural levels of vitamin D to increase. This is not a long-term fix, however, as the form of vitamin D the sun produces in our skin is different to the form you'll find in your health food store. The same is true of omega-3 in fish oil supplements versus omega-3 in fish. Whole foods in their natural form are always best.

I rarely use sunscreen anymore. I can't remember the last time my skin was burnt, and I tan easily. I don't do stupid things like hop on a plane in the middle of winter and then expect to be able to spend 10 hours a day in the tropical sun. I give my skin time to gradually adapt to sunlight, just as our ancestors would have done naturally from being outside as the seasons changed. The lower intensity of the sun in winter increases gradually during spring, ramping up that protective level of vitamin D to high levels by the time we're exposed to summer's intense sun. We modern-day humans still need daily sun exposure, often, and not just when we're on holiday. So go outside and get your solar panels under the sun!

Finding and Fixing the Mismatches

Sunlight is essential to our wellbeing. We evolved as creatures that lived in natural sunlight year round, within the cycles of day and night as well as seasonal shifts of longer and shorter days. Evolution gave us the means to capture sunlight and use it to power our physiological processes and to coordinate those processes using photoreceptors that drive our internal clocks. Our receptors are so sensitive they can tell the difference between morning, afternoon and evening sunlight.

We've created mismatches in the environment that prevent our circadian clocks from working as they should, disconnecting us from nature's cycles of light and darkness. We've created mismatches in our diet and lifestyle that have altered the ability of our body's solar panels to safely absorb the sunlight we need to power vitamin D production and many other critical body processes.

To fix this problem we need to realign our diet and lifestyle so it's closer to the lifestyle we were designed by evolution to thrive in. Here are ways to do that:

- Limit blue light exposure after darkness, getting to sleep between 9 pm and 11 pm each night.

- Sleep in a completely dark room.

- Eat early enough in the evening to allow at least two to three hours between finishing dinner and bedtime.

- Get your face directly into the sun the first thing upon rising (and not through glass).

- Get your skin and eyes exposed to morning and late afternoon sunlight as often as possible.

- Eat an ancestral diet that's rich in seafood.

- Stay adequately hydrated.

Here's another hint: If you eat a protein-rich breakfast within an hour of waking, you will have lasting energy well into the afternoon and it will help to reset your circadian clocks. Two benefits for the price of one!

We live in a blue-lit world, so completely blocking blue light in the evenings is a challenge, especially if you live in urban areas with 24-hour lighting or wish to have an evening social life. You can still light your environment with low-blue-light technology. F.lux (justgetflux.com) is a computer programme that can be downloaded for free to allow you to turn down most of the blue light on your computer screen. It will even set itself to automatically adjust your computer's level of blue light according to the time of your local sunrise and sunset.

There are blue-blocking screen protectors you can purchase for mobile phones and tablets. There are amber or low-blue-light bulbs you can get to replace the bright ones you may be using. And there are blue-blocker eyeglasses, varying from yellow to orange, that filter out the blue wavelengths of light. I use these glasses over my regular reading glasses in the evenings or by themselves when watching television after sunset. There is some modern technology we can use to more safely use other modern technology. We don't have to live in a cave to get the health benefits of living more like our ancestors!

A word about night-shift work. There isn't a fix. Night-shift work has been shown to be very detrimental to health over time, and now you can understand why. You can do your utmost to try to adapt your body to an unnatural circadian cycle, but you can't create true sunlight, which is what our bodies need, at night. You can only achieve a partial fix, at best, and your circadian clocks will become confused every time your shift changes. If you're a shift worker and your health is becoming compromised, you may need to change your job. That's the hard truth.

If you have filled out the Get Started Questionnaire, have a look at the questions around sleep, activities in the evening and your level of energy on awakening. Your answers should give you some information about how well your circadian clocks are working and what might be causing you problems. If you're struggling with obesity or cognitive decline, these are sure signs that your clocks are broken and need resetting. The suggestions listed above will give you a place to start resetting.

Biology always wins. It doesn't care about work deadlines or late-night social customs. It doesn't care that blue-lit computer and tablet screens are easier to see. It doesn't bend to our will when we try to extend our personal daylight into the night or switch our nights with our days in order to do a shift job.

We can align ourselves and recapture our health or we can suffer the consequences of our misalignments—it's our choice.

CHAPTER FIVE

Personal Magnetism

"If we continue to develop our technology without wisdom or prudence, our servant may prove to be our executioner." **OMAR N. BRADLEY**

There was a great debate in the science world in the early 1900s that changed the course of medicine, between two factions called 'vitalists' and 'physicalists'. For centuries, some theories about how the human body functioned could be lumped under the term 'vitalism', which claimed that there was a vital force, a 'life force', that organised and explained the physiological processes associated with human life. Treatment modalities—such as Traditional Chinese Medicine, acupuncture, Ayurvedic medicine, and homeopathy—that have been around for centuries and work with energy (like the Chinese Qi or Vedic prana) in some way, have this concept at their core. These 'alternative' forms of therapeutic treatment have remained in existence for so long because, quite simply, they produce results, whether or not the mechanism for those results is understood. (It's interesting how 'traditional' modalities became 'alternative', isn't it? But we won't go down that tunnel now.)

The other side of the debate, the physicalists' side, came about as a result of the discovery in the early 1900s that some organic chemical compounds were associated with physiological processes, thus beginning the science of biochemistry. The physicalists maintained that all physiological processes could be explained by biochemical reactions within the body. They considered vitalism to be superstitious bunk, and discredited vitalists and their theories. Biochemistry became the predominant focus of research and therapeutic treatment within the healthcare field, and it remains so today. This strikes me as a colossal example of throwing out the baby with the bathwater!

What happened as a result of the physicalists dominating the debate is that research focusing on energy or energy systems within the body (including light, electricity and magnetism) has been treated with scepticism, at best. At worst, many of those researchers were discredited and hounded out of academic positions. This lack of regard has continued to the present day, whenever new research threatens the hold biochemistry has on the healthcare sciences and their premise of better living through chemistry, one that fuels the pharmaceutical industry.

In reality, all that vitalists maintained was that there are physiological phenomena that cannot be explained by biochemical reactions alone. This is true—biochemistry actually cannot explain much about how the human body functions. This myopic view limits the focus of research and makes it unlikely that energy mechanisms will be researched in depth anytime soon. However, if we look through our evolutionary lens, we find that energy in its many forms explains a lot, including much about why we're getting sick and how we can help our bodies heal.

How We're Wired

To understand the concept of human beings as being electrically driven, we can go back to the work of Dr. Robert Becker, who I mentioned in the last chapter. Becker chose to work with salamanders to learn more about the natural electrical currents in the body because of a very special characteristic they possess: they can regenerate their limbs. If a limb is severed, the salamander simply grows a new one. Not only do they grow a new limb, they grow the correct limb. A severed left front leg is replaced by a regrown left front leg, not a right back leg. Many less complex organisms also have this ability, but as we humans evolved, this capacity was sacrificed for greater complexity—with one exception: We can regenerate bone. As an orthopaedic surgeon, Becker was understandably interested in how limbs heal. He searched for the signal that initiated the process of healing and discovered that it is not chemical but *electrical.* Score one for the vitalists!

Becker was able to measure subtle electrical currents passing between points along the salamanders' limbs that were not being transmitted by way of the nerves themselves. Instead, they appeared to follow what are known to many alternative practitioners as 'meridians' or lines of energy in the body. This occurs not only in salamanders, but in humans as well. We are, it appears, electromagnetic beings. Becker's book, *The Body Electric*, is very aptly named.

If electrical current is being transmitted throughout our bodies, you might be wondering what makes up the wiring along which the current is conducted. The answer is that a large part of our circuitry is made up of collagen, the substance most of us associate with the ligaments and tendons that hold our joints together and attach our muscles to the skeletal system. Collagen is located throughout the body, in all our tissues, and is especially abundant in the skin. In the last chapter you learned that the brain senses and responds to varying frequencies of light energy, and that our skin acts as a solar panel. We also have a vast and complex 'circuit board' within our bodies that allows the brain to send electrical signals to stimulate healing processes, such as bone regeneration.

It turns out that this internal wiring not only conducts electrical signals within the body but also *receives* signals from outside the body, much like a built-in GPS system. The GPS system in your car picks up wireless radio signals from a network of satellites orbiting the Earth, allowing the device to pinpoint your location and direct you to where you want to go. Our body's in-built GPS system uses the collagen network as a very sensitive antenna, allowing the body to receive electromagnetic signals from our environment. Those signals are then used to direct physiologic processes within the body. If "form follows function," then evolution must have had a purpose for creating this capability in us.

Listen to Your Mother (Earth, That Is...)

The term 'frequency' refers to the speed at which something pulses—high frequency means fast pulses, low frequency means slower pulses. The Earth gives off a natural low-frequency electromagnetic signal called the 'Schumann Resonance', which is powered by processes deep within the Earth's core, solar energy and lightning strikes around the globe. The strength of the Schumann Resonance's electromagnetic energy varies within the Earth's 24-hour light cycles, becoming more intense during daylight hours and less intense at night. Sensing these variations is another way that our bodies tell time.

We evolved within this ever-present pulsating signal, as did every other living thing on Earth. Furthermore, by evolution's design, we are all connected to this signal. The Schumann Resonance and the Earth's magnetic field make up the Earth's 'native electromagnetic field', or 'EMF'. We evolved within this ever-present field, and our ability to sense these native EMF signals is another way (along with light cycles) the body coordinates its processes. The body speaks in the language of frequencies and energy.

One of the surest ways we can connect with the Earth's electromagnetic signal is literally to connect with the Earth. We evolved over many thousands of years of putting our bare feet directly on the Earth, sleeping on the ground, putting our hands in the dirt, swimming in natural bodies of water—being in continuous physical connection with the Earth. Even when footwear began to be used, it was made of natural materials, such as animal skins, that are conductive.

In our modern world, we have broken our connection to that native electromagnetic field, by breaking our physical connection with the Earth. We wear shoes with soles made of unnatural insulating materials, such as synthetic rubber. We carpet our floors with artificial insulating fibres. We sleep off of the ground on raised beds and on insulating mattresses. We live in high-rise flats. We sit on synthetic fabric-covered furniture. We travel in vehicles that keep us raised up from the ground. All of this—and more—reduces our ability to sense and connect with the Earth's native EMF.

This disconnection from Mother Earth has a detrimental effect on our immune systems, increasing systemic inflammation and blocking the body's ability to access Becker's current of regeneration. The disconnection interferes with the body's ability to coordinate physiological processes. It also removes us from a source of free energy: electrons that can enter our bodies directly through our skin.

In Chapter Three I talked about how the fuel our body uses is electrons that come from our food—electrons that are stripped away from glucose or ketones within the mitochondria of our cells. These electrons get their energy from the sun and they form the current that flows through our bodies, providing the energy for all of our body processes. These electrons create the currents that flow through the body: the currents along the healing meridians Becker discovered, the currents that flip back and forth in the brain at night, the currents that cause the heart to beat, the currents that power every function in the body. Now you know that we have two sources of those electrons: the food we eat and direct contact with Mother Earth.

So, how do we get back in touch with the native electromagnetic field? The easiest and best way is through direct contact with the Earth, as we were designed by evolution to do.

The sole of the human foot has 1,300 nerve endings per square inch; more than any other surface of the body. There are no accidents with evolution. We were meant to connect, to place our bare feet on the ground. I recall watching the daughter of a friend who delighted in throwing off her shoes as she ran around in the grass, much to the consternation of her parents. I believe children discard their shoes because they feel better without them, because they pick up energy from the Earth. We need to learn to do the same.

Reconnecting with the Earth in this way doesn't need to be for the entire day. The more, the better—but even 20 to 30 minutes in the morning as you catch the morning sun would help. Or take your lunch break on a park bench and remove your shoes as you eat. When shoes are necessary, wear leather soles, because they provide some natural conductivity.

Other activities that can connect you to the Earth's EMF are swimming in outdoor bodies of water (avoid chlorinated pools) and gardening with your hands directly touching the soil. During times of the year when the weather limits direct contact with the Earth, you can use a grounding pad or grounding sheet. These can be purchased through online sources and used in your home. They facilitate a connection directly to the Earth, through a grounding rod or by using the grounding of your home's electrical system through an electrical outlet. Grounding shoes with conductive soles are now available for times when shoes must be worn.

Direct connection is always the best. Listen to your Mother: connect.

The Worst Smog Is the Kind You Can't See

The problem with antennae is that they pick up all kinds of signals, not just the ones you want them to. I used to make cross-country road trips in America in my car when I was younger, and I'd keep the radio on for company through the long hours. Those were the days before cassette tapes, CDs, and iPods. During a long trip, there would inevitably come a time when the station I was listening to started to fade and other radio signals would be picked up, interfering with my listening enjoyment. This happens in our bodies as well, because our sensitive collagen networks pick up electrical and magnetic signals from many different sources in our modern environment. These other signals are called 'non-native EMF'. They interfere with the body's listening enjoyment by swamping out the Earth's native EMF signals, flooding us with damaging signals instead.

Where do these non-native EMF signals come from? Non-native EMF sources from our technological world seem to be endless and growing. It all started with the introduction of electricity into our homes. Homes in the developed parts of the world tend to be electrically wired throughout. Current flows through our walls, ceilings and floors, and into our many electrical appliances. Whenever current flows, it generates magnetic fields as well. The problem is not really the flow of that electrical current itself as much as the irregular spikes that occur because of the current's *uneven* flow. This is known as 'dirty' electricity, and these spikes cause the greatest interference in our body's internal circuitry.

The worst non-native EMF players, though, are the many wireless devices used in our homes, neighbourhoods and cities. Mobile-phone masts send out radio waves that threaten to blanket the Earth. These towers are becoming so ubiquitous that I've found mobile phone reception in places as remote as the huge Maasai Mara Natural Reserve in Kenya.

Transmitters send radio signals to police and emergency services. Smart meters send regular, pulsed signals to utility companies so people don't have to come out to read meters. Broadband has brought Wi-Fi to most homes and businesses. These services are becoming so widespread that computers, tablets and smart phones can be used in most places on the globe. In populated areas, it's not uncommon to find 20 or more different Wi-Fi signals in any one location.

Microwaves are used in our kitchens and in the kitchens of most fast food restaurants. Our computers, tablets, smart phones and cordless phones not only receive electromagnetic signals, they also give off strong, pulsed signals.

We are living in a microwaved world, literally swimming in electromagnetic smog.

Non-native EMF can affect any system in the body, because the body depends on subtle electrical currents and electrical signals in order to function. These non-native fields disrupt the electrical signals our cells use to regulate all of our physiological functions. Cell membranes and the membranes surrounding our mitochondria are particularly affected, since they depend on a specific electrical potential across those membranes in order to function correctly. Mitochondrial membranes are many times more sensitive than cell membranes, and electromagnetic disruption of mitochondrial function negatively affects the way our cells produce energy, repair damaged proteins and regulate the growth and proliferation of new cells. An inability to repair damage and regulate growth is a prescription for cancer. Cancer cells have damaged mitochondria—they no longer function correctly and their growth is no longer checked.

There are devices available that allow you to 'see' this invisible electromagnetic smog. I encourage you to rent or buy such a device in order to check the status of your own particular environment. You'll need to be able to measure electric and magnetic fields, as well as microwaves. One such device is the reasonably priced TriField® Meter, which will pick up and measure a range of signals. You can purchase or rent devices that are even more sensitive, and technicians can be hired to check out your home and do the measurements for you. The strength of these fields drops off quickly with distance, as you'll see if you use a measuring device, so once you know where the 'hot' spots are, you can avoid the worst areas in your environment, or limit your time in them to help reduce their effects on your body.

The photo shows a TriField® Meter set to the magnetic scale (uppermost band) to measure non-native EMF from my laptop computer. You can see the needle pointing to nearly 10 milligauss, which is three times the upper safe limit. If I were to show you a video of this same setup, you would see the needle jumping back and forth, often pegging out at over 100 milligauss. The meter is sitting in the zone where my sensitive hands and wrists are located when I use the computer. These are also the exposures that my lap would be getting if I set my computer on it while I worked.

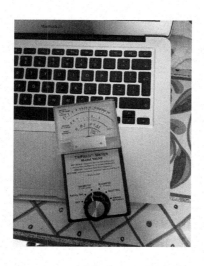

In the same way that we need to reconnect to the Earth, we also need to disconnect from our dependence on our non-native EMF devices. We may not be able to disconnect completely, because our modern world is becoming more and more computerised and wireless, making escape difficult. But we can limit our exposure and mitigate some of the damage. Turn off your Wi-Fi router at night. Even better, hardwire your computer into the router with a cable instead of using a wireless system. And find yourself an old corded phone. Go retro! When using your smart phone, use the speaker or a hands-free headset (but not a wireless one) and hold or carry your phone away from your body (rather than tucking it into your trouser pocket). Don't set your laptop on your lap and use it. Ground your computer (you can find easy instructions on the Internet about how to do this). Take all electrical devices out of your bedroom, including electric alarm clocks, TVs, mobile phones, chargers and electric blankets. Make your bedroom an electro-magnetic 'smog-free' zone to allow your body to heal at night. Also, refuse smart meters if they are offered by your utility company, and change smart meters over to standard meters wherever possible.

If you live in an area where the level of non-native EMF is high (which is pretty much any city) and where your ability to shield yourself is limited because of the many signals you can't control, you may need to move, particularly if your health is suffering. That is an inconvenient truth. The more you can reduce your exposure to non-native EMF and increase your exposure to the Earth's native field, the better your body is going to be able to heal and function as it was designed to.

Have a look at your Get Started Questionnaire and see what you have recorded for the amount of time you spend out-doors and the time of day. See also what you have recorded for your use of technology—the number of gadgets that you use, the hours of usage and the times during the day. This will give you an initial indication of your exposure to native and non-native EMF, and will point to some things that you can do to shift your environment and your habits in order to minimise the former and maximise the latter.

Biology always wins. It doesn't care whether you can receive your emails round the clock from any location. It doesn't care whether you can find that location without a map. Biology doesn't care if you find it inconvenient to slowly cook your food or to wind your clock or to stand in one place to have a telephone conversation. Human biology evolved in a non-technological world. We're designed to respond to our environment by altering the way our body functions, doing so by epigenetically switching our genes on and off. We need to turn off the technological switches in our environment in order to allow our body's epigenetic switches to be favourably set for healing.

CHAPTER SIX

A Thirst for Life

"Natural forces within us are the true healers of disease." **HIPPOCRATES**

Before we get into the meat of this chapter, let's review what we know so far. We know that our bodies are like hybrid cars: We run on two different fuels—glucose and ketones—and both ultimately do the same thing; they deliver electrons to our mitochondria, those little engines within all our cells that power our physiological processes. Those electrons get their energy from the sun. We also know that there's a source of free energy—in the form of electrons—that enters our bodies directly through our skin when we make contact with the Earth. We know that we have complex circuitry made up of collagen 'wires' that carry electrical signals from one part of the body to another, including the signals necessary for regeneration and healing. We know that our collagen network also receives signals from our outside environment—it receives healing and regulating signals from the Earth and disruptive, damaging signals from our technological devices. We also know that we receive light signals from the sun that allow our biological clocks to synchronize so that we can sleep, regenerate, make new memories, regulate our fat stores and heal at night.

But there's one big piece we haven't explored yet, and that's how to charge our batteries. That's what this chapter is about.

Charging Your Body Battery

A battery has two functions: storing an electrical charge and driving an electrical current. When you use a battery for a torch (that's a 'flashlight' for you Yanks), you can see that it has two different ends, one that's positively charged (+) and one that's negatively charged (-). When you put the battery into the torch and turn it on, current flows from one end of the battery, through the light bulb, to the other end of the battery, to create light. The current is made up of electrons that energise the materials in the light bulb. When the battery's charge runs out, it can no longer push the electrons through the circuit. At that point, we throw the battery away and replace it. Our 'body battery' isn't the disposable kind, however.

What is our body battery made of? Our battery is more like the one in my first car. That battery was an older type, the kind I had to put water in, along with something called 'electrolyte solution' to allow the battery to hold its charge. If the water was low or if there wasn't enough electrolyte solution, the battery would weaken and run down easily, even though it was being charged by the engine. For the battery to work, it needed to be continually charged *and* to have the capacity to hold that charge. This is the type of battery the human body has.

You may be surprised at what our battery is made of: water, DHA (a special type of Omega-3 fatty acid) and sunlight.

The water in our bodies allows us to hold a charge and to drive electrical currents throughout our collagen wire network. Our body is filled with water. It's in all of our cells, in the spaces between our cells, and it makes up most of our blood, 85% of brain matter and 75% of our overall volume. It's common knowledge that we can go for some time without food but can't function for long without water. Our systems simply shut down during severe dehydration. This wasn't fully understood until the recent discovery of some of water's amazing properties.

It's been known for centuries that water can be found in three phases: solid (in the form of ice), liquid or gas (as vapour or steam). Gerald Pollack, in his book *The Fourth Phase of Water,* describes the discovery of a new phase of water—one in which the water molecules line up in a structured lattice, as they would in a solid substance, but the molecules are *also* free-flowing, as they would be in a liquid phase. This, in itself, is interesting, but it's the unique electrical properties of this phase of water that make the discovery astounding.

It's worth explaining that some substances are attracted to water (they're called 'hydrophilic') and others are repelled by water ('hydrophobic'). An example of a hydrophobic substance is oil. We know it's difficult to get oil and water to mix, and it's because of oil's water-repelling property. An example of a hydrophilic substance is—wait for it—collagen!

Water likes to cosy up to collagen, and that's where the magic happens. When water comes into contact with collagen, it forms the newly discovered type of water (structured *and* free-flowing) in a zone adjacent to the surface of the collagen. This zone is called an 'exclusion zone', or EZ, because when the water molecules take on a structured form, they squeeze out any substances that are dissolved in the water. The most magical thing is that the EZ pushes water's positive charges to one side and its negative charges to the other side and drives an electrical current through the middle. In other words—it creates a battery! All through our bodies, water-loving proteins like collagen come into contact with water. This gives the body its ability to store charges and push electrical currents. Is it any wonder that we lose energy—or even die—when we become dehydrated? Dehydration takes away our battery. No more current, no more life!

DHA is another ingredient of the body's battery. DHA is a special type of omega-3 fatty acid found in high concentrations in marine animals like shellfish, salmon, mackerel, sardines and other oily fish. DHA is like the electrolyte solution that allowed that old battery in my car to hold its charge. DHA is unique among the fatty acids for its ability to capture and hold electrons. No other type of fat does it in the same way. This is why the brain, our biggest energy hog, is loaded with DHA. It's loaded, that is, only if we have enough DHA in our diets, since the body can't produce it in any appreciable amount. This is why seafood is at the top of the list of preferred foods (as stated in Chapter Three). Without DHA, our battery is hampered in its ability to hold a charge.

So, how does our water-collagen-DHA-battery get charged? Sunlight! In Pollack's experiments, he noticed that the formation of the exclusion zone at the surface of a protein (like collagen) was affected by light, specifically infrared light and ultraviolet light. Both are components of sunlight. Infrared light is the part of sunlight that gives it its warmth. When the EZ is exposed to infrared light, it expands, making a bigger battery. And when the EZ is exposed to ultraviolet rays, it gets more energised and drives more current. Sunlight makes the body's battery bigger and more powerful.

If you didn't have enough reasons to get out in the sunlight already, this should convince you! The interaction of water, sunlight and DHA has provided the perfect template for evolution to construct organisms as complex and energy-demanding as mammals (including us). If you didn't already have enough reasons to reduce your exposure to blue light, here's another one: excessive blue light destroys DHA.

How Our Cells Communicate: Water Memory

Our body speaks in the language of frequencies and wavelengths. Light has frequencies and wavelengths; electromagnetic fields also have frequencies and wavelengths. It turns out that biochemical reactions may also rely on frequencies and wavelengths—if we view them from a new perspective.

One of the ways the body initiates reactions is when a protein stimulates a receptor. For example, our body is full of different hormones that have corresponding receptors that are sensitive to those hormones. This is sometimes described as a type of lock and key system, with the hormone as the 'key' that fits into the receptor's 'lock'. Opening the lock sets a biological process in motion. Earlier in this book, we looked at the hormone leptin and how it stimulates leptin receptors in the hypothalamus, our brain's bean-counter, setting in motion either fat-burning or fat-storing. We also looked at vitamin D and how every tissue in the body has vitamin D receptors that set a wide range of processes in motion when unlocked.

One of the enigmas, though, has been how a hormone manages to find its receptor within a cell. A hormone is just a protein. It doesn't have fins and can't propel itself, so it relies on another means of locomotion. There's a phenomenon called 'Brownian motion'. It occurs when molecules move around simply by bumping into and bouncing off of other molecules. The result is random movement. A hormone protein randomly hitting a receptor within a cell is a bit like a speck of dust in your drawing room randomly finding its way to one particular spot on one of your walls. The probability is practically nil. You wouldn't want to pay much for that lottery ticket!

A theory about how proteins and receptors 'talk' to each other and find each other without being in direct contact is linked to another special property of water. A renowned French scientist by the name of Jacques Benveniste stumbled upon an interesting phenomenon when he added biological substances to water. One of those substances was a particular antibody (a protein made by the body) that interacts with a specific type of white blood cell during some types of immune reactions. Benveniste added the antibody to pure water and then diluted that antibody solution many times over—to the point where, statistically, there would be no chance of any of the antibody being left in the solution. What he discovered was that the diluted solution behaved in the same way as the original antibody: It stimulated an immune reaction. Those experiments were repeated with other biological agents and duplicated in laboratories in four countries, with the same results. It was as if the water 'remembered' the substance that had been dissolved in it. This phenomenon became known as 'water memory'.

That experiment's process of serial dilution is the same process homeopaths use to prepare their solutions. They perform a series of dilutions until the original material is gone, and the resulting substance is used to stimulate a healing response. Homeopaths consider 'water memory' to be proof of the science behind homeopathy.

Though Benveniste was not trying to prove anything about homeopathy, you might imagine the uproar his experiments caused when he published his results in 1988 in the journal *Nature*. There's a long story behind what happened, but the end result was that Benveniste was publicly ridiculed, lost his funding, lost his research programme and lost his reputation as a researcher. Water memory became a joke within the scientific community, and research of this nature was significantly set back. Score one for the physicalists!

In spite of his rejection, Benveniste spent the rest of his life continuing his experiments, searching for the mechanism behind water memory. It was already known that molecules emit detectable electromagnetic signals and that the frequencies of those signals are unique to each molecule, acting like a sort of 'electromagnetic fingerprint'. Benveniste hypothesized that water was able to pick up that unique molecular signal and re-transmit the signal, even when the original substance had gone. That implied that a biological key does not need to be in direct contact with its receptor, because it can 'telegraph' its message through water.

Along came another French scientist, this one by the name of Luc Montagnier (he won a Nobel Prize for his discovery of the HIV virus, which puts him up there in the league of great scientists). Montagnier was familiar with the work of Benveniste and was interested in the energy-transmission properties of water as a possible explanation for Benveniste's results. He knew that molecules transmit unique electromagnetic signals and that electromagnetic signals can travel long distances through many materials, so he set up an experiment to test whether or not a 'long-distance' molecular signal could stimulate a specific reaction.

Montagnier put two test tubes of purified water in close proximity to one another. In one test tube, he put a fragment of DNA and in the second test tube he put fragments of the materials that make up DNA. What he discovered was that in the second test tube, the fragments assembled themselves into a strand of DNA identical to the one in the first test tube. The electromagnetic signal was transmitted not only through the water but across the space between the test tubes as well!

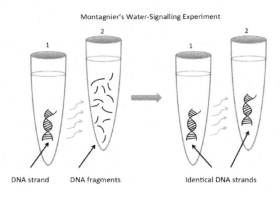

Montagnier's Water-Signalling Experiment

DNA strand   DNA fragments   Identical DNA strands

Although Montagnier's experiments have since been reproduced by other laboratories, his results were met with disbelief and criticism, similar to the way Benveniste's experiments were received. Today, much to the Western scientific community's loss, Montagnier now conducts his research in China, where he's found greater openness to research that challenges our current understanding of biological interactions.

What does all of this have to do with health and chronic illness? Well, in addition to now knowing that, as Luc Montagnier maintains, "High dilutions of something are not nothing", and that homeopathy may indeed have a scientific basis, the discoveries I've told you about in this chapter offer three other very important implications for our health.

The first is the most obvious: We need water, and lots of it, in order for our bodies to communicate in the language of frequencies and give the commands needed to regulate biological processes. Not enough water equals not enough communication.

Second, if water can pick up and transmit subtle electro-magnetic signals of the regulating proteins, like hormones, then guess what else it can pick up and transmit? You guessed it: modern-day electromagnetic smog! Too much environmental interference crowding the body's recep-tors means we can't really tune in to our natural, molecular 'radio stations' very well.

And, third, measurements of the electromagnetic signals emitted from molecules have shown that *molecular shape matters*. If the shape of a molecule changes, even if its chem-ical make-up stays the same, that molecule will send out a different signal. This may begin to explain why there's a link between misshapen or 'bent' proteins and Alzheimer's or Parkinson's Disease. Bent proteins give off a different signal, one that is, at best, ineffective and, at worst, damaging. This is why trans fats are so damaging to the body—they embed themselves into our cell membranes and block the normal signalling within those membranes.

The importance of molecular shape is also why supplements don't take the place of nature's versions of the nutrients our body needs. The vitamin D in a supplement is not the same shape as the vitamin D our body manufactures. The DHA in fish oil supplements is not the same shape as the DHA in seafood, due to the shape-altering effects of the extraction process. Just because a supplement has the same chemical composition as its natural cousin does not mean that it behaves the same way. The lesson is that if our body is designed to produce it, we should let it. And if we need to get what the body needs from food sources, we need to eat real food.

How Much Is Enough?

It's safe to say that the majority of people in the Western world go around with some level of dehydration for much, if not most, of the time—even those who drink litres of water each day. Part of the reason for this is the dehydrating nature of our carb-loaded Western diet, which demands more water to metabolise. An even bigger reason is that non-native EMF breaks down water within our cells. It literally dehydrates us. This is why you can't drink yourself out of dehydration when you're in an environment loaded with electromagnetic smog.

One of the ways we can evaluate our level of cellular hydration is through some simple blood tests that are part of the routine suite of blood tests commonly done when you have your periodic health check-up. It turns out that the ratio of an analyte called 'blood urea nitrogen', or BUN, and another analyte called 'creatinine' is an indicator of cellular hydration. If the ratio of BUN to creatinine is ten or below (where BUN and creatinine are measured in mg/dL), it's a good sign. Any higher indicates some level of dehydration. It also means that your battery is weak. (In the UK, we use different units and measure 'urea' instead of BUN: Divide urea in mmol/L by creatinine in umol/L and then divide the result by 0.00403. If the resulting number is ten or below, it's a good sign; higher indicates dehydration.)

I've been drinking between two and three litres of water a day for years now, regardless of whether or not I'm thirsty. Yet I have struggled to get my BUN-to-creatinine ratio down to the ideal level. I've gotten close, primarily by doing all of the things listed in the last chapter to reduce my exposure to non-native EMF and to get more grounded to the Earth. I look forward to seeing how much better things will get now that I've moved away from the city.

Water is crucial. It's needed for cellular signalling and for our metabolic processes. Water facilitates fat metabolism.

Water is needed for forming our body's battery, for transmitting healing electrical currents, for all of the thousands of biological processes that our body undergoes every day.

With chronic dehydration, we become disconnected from our thirst signal, so we may need to consciously choose to drink more until we become sensitive to our body's water needs again.

Quality Matters

If push comes to shove, drinking poor-quality water is better than not drinking enough water. That said, the quality of the water we drink matters greatly. Part of the water-quality issue has to do with contaminants. Our water treatment processes leave a lot of compounds in the water, including things like antibiotics and oestrogens from birth control pills. These compounds make their way through the sewage treatment process into surface water and, from there, to the water treatment plants, where they are not fully removed. While such contaminants are present in small concentrations, ingesting small concentrations over time does have an impact. And then there are the BPA (bisphenol A) compounds that leach into bottled water from plastic containers, and which act as oestrogen-like substances in our bodies. All of these 'oestrogenic' substances are 'endocrine disruptors', meaning they disrupt our hormone balances.

As if *that* isn't enough bad news, one of the worst players in this drama of water quality is fluoride. Fluoridation of municipal water supplies is widespread in America. Although most of Europe has, so far, resisted this practice, in the UK there is a big push to fluoridate all of the country's municipal water supplies. The main argument for doing so is to prevent tooth decay. A better way to prevent tooth decay might be to reduce the level of dietary sugar that's causing the tooth decay in the first place. Fluoride does not have to be ingested in order to negatively affect the body's processes; skin absorption can have an affect as well. That's enough to ruin a lovely shower!

When fluoride exposure is high—or lower but the exposure continues over time—it accumulates in bones and teeth, causing structural abnormalities in bones and damage to tooth enamel. Fluoride also blocks iodine receptors in the body because of their similar atomic behaviour. Every tissue in our body has iodine receptors, and evolution doesn't design anything that has no function. The thyroid gland acts as the accelerator for our metabolism, so when the brain wants to raise our metabolic rate, it signals the thyroid gland to jack up the engines. That process depends on iodine (yet another good reason to make sure seafood is high on the list of foods to include in our diet). But if our iodine receptors are blocked by fluoride, our metabolism can't function effectively. Thyroid disease, particularly hypothyroidism, is skyrocketing in the Western world, and fluoride toxicity is believed to be a large contributor.

The biggest issue with fluoride, however, has to do with our body's bioelectric properties, which, as you probably realise by now, are critical to life. Our collagen wire network must be able to conduct electrical currents. Fluoride is a 'dielectric blocker'. For you non-geeks, that means fluoride blocks the flow of electrical currents in the body. This is big-time bad news. Fluoride is one of those substances that manages to cross the blood-brain barrier—the protective barrier that keeps most things that circulate through our bloodstream away from our delicate brain tissue—meaning that fluoride also blocks the currents in our brains.

What can we do about this? First, we need to be hydrating ourselves with good-quality water. If you have a fluoridated municipal water supply, you will need to find another source of water for drinking and cooking. Boiling and ordinary filtering do not remove fluoride. The only kind of filter that removes fluoride is a 'reverse osmosis filter'. They are expensive and can be problematic to maintain, but they are certainly an option. However, it may be more cost-effective simply to buy good bottled water. You want the water you buy to be in glass bottles, not plastic, because of the BPA problem. Spring water, mineral water, well water, reverse-osmosis-treated water—those are all good options. Watch out for bottled water that comes from a municipal water source, as you could just be buying the same fluoride problem.

Have a look at your Get Started Questionnaire and see what you've listed for your water intake amount and the source of your water. You can also look at your use of technology to see how your environment may be dehydrating you even if your water intake is sufficient. If you've had a recent blood test that included BUN (or urea) and creatinine levels, you can do the calculation to see how dehydrated you may be. Dehydration means that your battery is weak.

Biology always wins. It doesn't care if it's easier to load our water supply with fluoride than to stop feeding our children sugar. It doesn't care if it costs you more to find good-quality water and good-quality food. Biology needs what it needs, irrespective of how you choose to spend your money. For biology, good quality water is not a luxury—it's an imperative. Either we pay now, or we pay in increased ill health and physical degeneration later. We choose to align with our evolutionary biology or we choose the consequences—it's as straightforward as that.

The good news is that we have a say in whether or not we move down the spiral into chronic disease, early ageing and spending the latter part of life fighting a battle of deterioration of body and mind. There is room for choice here, and that is the greatest hope the information in this book provides. The direction your body and your health is heading is not written in stone, and it's never too late to start turning things around and heading in a healthy direction.

CHAPTER SEVEN

Blocks and Levers

"Everything can be taken from a man but one thing: the last of human freedoms—to choose one's attitude in any given set of circumstances, to choose one's own way." **VIKTOR E. FRANKL**

One thing you can be sure of as you embark on any change is that you will encounter resistance—from within as well as from without. We get comfortable with the way things are, even when we don't like the way things are, because the unknown alternative gives our imaginative minds a lot to work with.

A second thing you can be sure of is that the resistance you encounter is going to be in direct proportion to the size of the change. Changing the time that you eat lunch would probably cause nothing more than minor irritation, if that. But if you change something like your job, your social activities, where you live or even what you eat, you can expect massive resistance to emerge. You may even have already experienced some of that resistance as you've read through this book and come across some things you may need to change if you're going to recover your health. ("You mean

I'll have to do *that*?!")

A third thing you can be sure of is that the volume of the resistance will get louder if other people are involved in the changes you're making, whether they're directly affected or simply interested in what you're doing. Recall what I said about my own journey and the difficulty I encountered while climbing out of the conventional wisdom soup bowl. If I hadn't overcome that resistance, I would still be floating in it and, no doubt, getting sicker. But I got out, and so can you.

In previous chapters we've looked at environments we've created that are out of alignment with how our bodies have been designed over hundreds of thousands of years of evolution to function. We've also looked at ways we can realign our environments to enable our bodies to heal and thrive. Realignment is change, and some of those realigning changes will, most likely, need to be substantial. That means you may affect other people as you embark on a new path to a healthy future. You can't have your Neolithic cake and your health, too!

This chapter is focused on identifying resistance and roadblocks you may encounter, and what you can do about them. It also suggests ways of finding allies in your quest for greater health and vitality.

Let's start with the blocks in our own heads, because positively affecting all the other blocks—including our ability to find allies—hinges on addressing our internal blocks.

The Power of Thought: Mind Over Matter and the Placebo Effect

First of all, it's very helpful to believe that a future without chronic, debilitating illness and early ageing is even possible for us. There's ample data to show that the mind has a powerful affect on the body, and not only because of its impact on our emotions and our emotions' impact on our physiology. Our thoughts measurably affect our physiological processes.

Dr. Lissa Rankin, in her book *Mind Over Medicine,* examines the phenomenon called the 'placebo effect', in which a person is given a 'fake', innocuous medicine or procedure and has a healing response *simply because they believe that the drug or procedure was real.* The fake drug or procedure is called a 'placebo'. In randomised controlled trials for testing new drugs, one group of subjects is given the real drug and another group is given the placebo. In double-blind tests, neither the researchers administering the drugs nor the recipients know whether the drug is real. In order for a new drug to qualify as effective, the drug must do better than a placebo in delivering beneficial results. Rankin notes that some studies demonstrated that test groups receiving the placebo drug or fake procedure sometimes fared *better* than those who received the real thing.

The attitude of the majority of the medical research world is to dismiss the placebo effect as nothing ("It's all in the mind"). Yes, it is all in the mind! So, what does this tell us about the power of the mind and the power of the body to repair itself? And why is that power not being leveraged to help patients to heal?

The placebo effect can work the opposite way. Cancer patients are told they have a specific number of months to live and are advised to go put their affairs in order. Patients suffering from Type 2 diabetes are told that they'll eventually get worse and need insulin. Patients with mild cognitive impairment are told it will eventually lead to full-blown dementia. All of these messages are invitations for patients to live into those realities, which they often do (called the 'nocebo effect').

It appears that belief alone can create physical changes in the body. The placebo effect is not nothing. If evolution did design internal healing systems within our body, the mind evidently plays a part in whether or not the body accesses and engages those systems.

Recall that the first important event that caused my downward-spiralling health to reverse course was the intervention of a Traditional Chinese Medicine practitioner who helped me stop seeing Alzheimer's Disease as a foregone conclusion in my life. I changed my beliefs and that opened a door to a new possibility. I can't say for certain that Alzheimer's is not on my horizon, but it isn't here now. Without that shift in my thinking, I'd quite likely have ensured that it would manifest. Reversing disease, or the likelihood of it, began with changing my beliefs and then my behaviours.

We have the capacity to think ourselves sick and to think ourselves well. I don't think this means you can do damaging things to your body and then get off scot-free by simply believing they will do no harm. The evidence of this is our widespread delusion that we can continue to live as we're living in our Western societies and avoid the healthcare crisis we're now facing.

The change in action that's needed begins with a change in beliefs. The first belief to change is that reversing chronic illness is possible. Then there are things we can do to put that reversal in motion. Thoughts have the ability to create our reality in ways the body evidently responds to.

I've spent the past 18 years as a transformational trainer for businesses, organisations and in the public sector, teaching the skills of Attitudinal Intelligence™. This methodology, developed by Dr. K. Bradford Brown, is based on recognizing that our attitudes are formed from our beliefs about ourselves, others and the situations we're in, and that those beliefs are often untrue and unchallenged. Further, those attitudes influence our emotions and drive our behaviours.

For example, when I saw what was happening to members of my family regarding their declining health, I began to believe that I was next on the list for early-onset dementia, especially when I started experiencing cognitive glitches. Based on my early research and conversations with health professionals, I came to believe that there was no way of stopping the process and no cure. My beliefs coalesced into an attitude of hopelessness and resignation about my fate and my future. That attitude generated behaviours, such as not talking to others about what I was experiencing and not considering taking opportunities that required a lengthy time investment, because I 'knew' I wouldn't have all my marbles long enough to make them worth the effort.

Beliefs beget attitudes beget behaviours. I had to change my beliefs before I could begin to look for solutions.

Inconvenient Truths

Once you've done the thought work to get past your initial blocking beliefs and you've leapt into action, you'll need to address other kinds of resistance that may emerge. Here's a taste of what some of that resistance might sound like in your head:

- "I'll look silly wearing those yellow glasses, and it makes the television screen look a different colour."

- "It's such a pain to have to turn off the router every night and then re-boot it in the morning."

- "Organic foods are so much more expensive, and they don't last as long. It's probably just a ploy to make us pay more."

- "I'm naturally a night owl. I can't just change my nature now."

- "If it was only me who changed, that would be okay, but I can't inconvenience my family."

- "These new ways of doing things are making my family complain, and I don't know if it's worth it."

- "Other people matter more than I do."

- "I need to be sure this is going to make a difference before I try it."

- "I'm too old to change my ways."

- "People are going to think I'm crazy and ridicule me."

- "I'll lose touch with the world if I have to give up my technology."

- "I'll never be able to go out with my friends at night or go on holidays again."

Remember my repeated statements about biology always winning? How biology doesn't care whether things are convenient or acceptable to our friends and family or whether the best thing for our body is the cheapest option? Developing and using technology to create convenience is part of what got us into this pickle in the first place!

All of this new information about how our body really functions in connection with our environment amounts to a stack of inconvenient truths—if we view it from a perspective of being wedded to our modern way of life. From another perspective, this new information amounts to a hopeful, liberating prescription for living a vibrant, healthy life well into old age. *Same situation, different attitude.* The first perspective will trip you up at every challenge; the other will provide you with your body's North Star and the courage to head toward it, no matter what.

You need to make *you* matter the most when it comes to your health and your future, because you're not much good to anyone else if you don't. You are the one who has the most at stake and the most to lose if you continue to create and live in an environment that goes against your biology as it has evolved. Once you decide that you matter and that you're worth the investment for a healthier future, all sorts of new possibilities open up, and the task of finding new creative ways to do things becomes an adventure.

Here are some examples of situations and how switching perspectives can make change easier.

Eating at a restaurant. On a night out at a restaurant, instead of looking at the menu through the lens of "Look at all the things I can't eat!" try asking yourself, "What can I choose and/or what can I substitute that will enhance my health?" Most restaurants are aware of and accommodating of a variety of dietary needs these days (such as gluten sensitivity) and are happy to let you make substitutions, usually at no extra cost. I've often asked to substitute some wilted spinach for potatoes on my breakfast plate, or to have extra vegetables instead of rice or potatoes on my dinner plate. I can't recall a single time my request was refused. I simply tell the waiter I can't eat the item for health reasons, and it's no problem. In some dining-out situations, you might need to take along foods for yourself or even eat something before you go out.

Wearing blue-blocker lenses in public. I'll soon be attending a three-day summit in America, one that will have sessions that extend into the evenings. You can be sure I'll have my blue-blocker lenses on once the sun has set, in order to cut out the blue light, especially since the time zone difference will have disturbed my usual circadian rhythms. My glasses will no doubt stimulate questions, but that gives me opportunities to tell others about the dangers of blue light toxicity. Spreading the word is one of my missions, after all. Explaining about my odd glasses makes for very interesting conversations and is a great ice-breaker!

In the sun and on the ground. Finding ways to get into the sun and get your feet in contact with the ground can be another challenge. View it as an opportunity for connection and adventure. Take a few minutes each day to watch sunrises and sunsets. This will not only improve your physical health, but your mental health as well. Roll in the grass with your children. Wear leather shoes or walk with bare feet when you take your dog for a walk. Even doing small things will soon have you becoming more aware of how light changes throughout the days and the seasons while you gather in those free electrons from direct contact with the Earth. Hug a tree every chance you get. Really! It will do more than help you get grounded; being around trees gives you the opportunity to breathe in all the oxygen trees give off (especially pine trees).

What If People Think You're Looney Tunes?

How do you handle people looking at you funny, thinking you're bonkers, offering unhelpful advice or refusing to support you in your efforts?

This is where having your own attitude squared away and knowing why you're making the changes you're making will help you immensely. There's nothing like being true to your purpose internally to make the example you're setting catch people's attention. Your results will speak for themselves. That, more than anything else, will get others on board with what you're doing. You are the person with the most at stake regarding your health, though, so you get to call the shots about your own body. Full stop. But other people get to call the shots about their own bodies, as well, so no preaching. We each choose our own path, and preaching about yours will only get up the other person's nose and not help your case. Let them be curious, and give them information if they ask for it. That will help you build allies.

Getting your health practitioner on board with your efforts may or may not be easy. It depends on how open he or she is to ideas beyond those they were taught in medical school. I shared what I was doing with my GP and she helped me where she could, within the limits of what the National Health Service permitted. This allowed me to take charge of my own health while getting some support when I needed it. You may find, however, that your physician is not willing to be a consultant on your journey or is dismissive about what you're doing regarding your health. In that case, you may need to change doctors to find one who's more willing to work with you in partnership. You are always in charge of decisions about your health.

You're likely to find unhelpful conventional wisdom coming out of the mouths of your family and friends. One would hope that they have your best interests at heart and have good intentions, even if their suggestions are misguided. It's up to you to take a stand about what you need and to ask them to support you in your efforts to turn your health around. Some of the most sceptical people in your life may shift their own attitudes as they see the results you're getting by making changes.

Connecting via online sites and social media is a way to find like-minded people who are making some of the same changes you're making. I include a few websites and social media sites in the resources section at the end of the book. I hesitate to refer you to online sites as a resource—only because getting online is both a blessing and a curse, as it comes with a dose of non-native EMF and blue light. But if you are discerning about how and when you use the computer, the Internet can be a very helpful resource.

There are other resources to help you work with the beliefs and attitudes that may be getting in the way of your ability to make changes and stick with them in the face of push-back from others or resistance from within. The More To Life Programme (www.moretolife.org) offers public courses that teach skills for uncovering and powerfully changing limiting beliefs. And in my workshops and coaching I help participants and clients recognise and break through the mental and emotional roadblocks that get in the way of their efforts to create a pathway to health.

For me, the biggest roadblocks on my path to reversing illness have always been of my own making. Even when others don't get on board with what I'm doing, I know that I'm free to choose how I respond and to make my own choices for my own health. To paraphrase Viktor Frankl: The one freedom that can't be taken from us is the ability to choose our attitude. That extends to choosing our own path.

CHAPTER EIGHT

Conclusions

"Learn from yesterday, live for today, hope for tomorrow. The important thing is not to stop questioning."

ALBERT EINSTEIN

Humans evolved within an environment of natural rhythms, in connection to the Earth, exposed to the sun, eating foods produced naturally, drinking water from natural sources. Our bodies were designed through evolutionary processes to sensitively respond to environmental cues from all of those different sources in order to ensure our survival. In harmony with natural forces, we're wired for health and healing.

But we no longer live in the world of our Paleolithic ancestors, or even the world I grew up in. Over only a few decades, technology has altered our landscapes, water quality, oceans, food sources, air, night skies, connection to the Earth and even the intensity of the sunlight, due to our affect on the ozone layer. This all means that if we want our health and vitality back we can't simply revert to eating as our ancestors did. We must do more.

In this book, I've presented the foundation of a new paradigm based on a wealth of new research about how the human body functions in response to its environment. I've attempted to present the big picture by distilling and translating a great deal of information down to the basics, connecting various pieces of the puzzle that this new research is uncovering. Other people are connecting pieces of the puzzle in a much deeper and more thorough way. What's in this book is only the tip of the iceberg—but it's a big tip of a big iceberg. Even becoming familiar with this tip, as presented in this book, can help you create a significantly healthier future for yourself.

Adopting this new paradigm will allow you to use an evolutionary lens to uncover the ways the modern environment—and your particular environment—is misaligned with the way your body was designed by evolution to function and heal.

To recover your health and vitality, you'll need to become an evolutionary sleuth, searching your own environment for misalignments in the four key areas of diet, light, electromagnetism and water. The Get Started Questionnaire (which you can access here: evolutionaryreboot.com/get-started-questionnaire) will give you data to work with about elements of your current environment and how you're responding to them; elements such as your diet, your sleeping patterns, your activities, your use of technology, your energy and your mood. The information in this book shows you where to aim your magnifying glass and what to do about the misalignments you find. When you've identified your misalignments, you can use the information in this book to correct them, if possible; mitigate them, where correction isn't possible; and thus redirect the course of your health. Start searching, Sherlock!

Don't Complicate Things

The science behind the way our modern-day environment is degrading our health is complex, but the ways to fix it don't have to be. For example, eating whole foods that have been naturally grown or raised doesn't have to be complicated. It doesn't involve counting calories or macronutrients, and there's no weighing of portions—only applying some common sense. Does the food you want to eat grow naturally in the region where you live? Is it in season? If your answers are yes and yes, then go for it. If not, it's best to leave it alone, even if there's a transition time involved as you figure things out. Does a food item come with a list of unpronounceable ingredients? Then give it a miss. As you find more and more food items that are good for you, you can leverage modern technology by buying in bulk and having them delivered to your door!

Getting some direct exposure to sunlight every day doesn't need to be complicated either. Nor does putting your bare feet onto the grass (or with leather-soled shoes). Turning off your gadgets at night and taking them all the way out of your bedroom before going to sleep is also not complicated.

Putting on a pair of blue-blocker glasses to minimise your blue light exposure is not complicated. Finding a source of good water does not have to be complicated. You might be surprised, as you begin to explore solutions, how easy it's going to be to make changes.

This is not to say that it won't take *some* effort on your part. It will. You'll likely find that some of the changes you want to make to correct the misalignments are inconvenient. In our technological world, we've been trading our health for convenience. It's time to reverse that swap and trade convenience for our health. When you get over being irritated at the inconvenience of making your lifestyle healthier in these ways, you may find that what takes its place was worth the effort: newfound joy and energy, vastly improved health, connection to the world around you and to others and a sense of liberation that comes from knowing that you have new choices and possibilities for your health. Trading some convenience for those results becomes a no-brainer.

Making the changes stick will require some patience. It has likely taken years of living in a certain way to get you to where you are today, so you won't reverse everything overnight. Depending on how much damage has been done to your systems and what your current environmental conditions are, you may not be able to reverse everything. But any of your circumstances can be improved.

For example, if you're diabetic and dependent on insulin, you may not be able to repair the beta cells in your pancreas if they're too far gone, but you can greatly improve your blood sugar regulation, and you can side-step or repair other conditions associated with having diabetes, like damage to your peripheral nerves. This could add years and quality to your life.

I have an autoimmune condition that causes my body to attack my thyroid gland, making me hypothyroid. I don't know if too much damage has been done for my thyroid to function on its own again without medication, but I am actively reversing the systemic inflammation by making changes in my environment to prevent any further damage. And I'll see how it goes.

Making these changes in your lifestyle and your environment will require you to be bold enough to act on your own behalf and committed enough to keep going when your own mind or other people create roadblocks. You can, and you need to, become your own best advocate, because it's you who has the most to lose if you don't. And the most to gain if you do.

You can address the changes one at a time, layering them into your daily life as you add each one. Or you can do a deep dive and make a lot of changes at once. Whichever route you go, take notes, monitor your progress and notice how your body responds as you realign with your evolutionary origins. The main thing is to begin somewhere. Just start. Motion begets motion.

This passage from W. H. Murray in *The Scottish Himalaya Expedition* may inspire you:

"Until one is committed, there is hesitancy, the chance to draw back, always ineffectiveness. Concerning all acts of initiative (and creation), there is one elementary truth, the ignorance of which kills countless ideas and splendid plans: that the moment one definitely commits oneself, the providence moves too. All sorts of things occur to help one that would never otherwise have occurred. A whole stream of events issues from the decision, raising in one's favor all manner of unforeseen incidents and meetings and material assistance, which no man could have dreamt would have come his way. I learned a deep respect for one of Goethe's couplets: 'Whatever you can do, or dream you can do, begin it. / Boldness has genius, power, and magic in it!'"

Share Your Success

A great way to find and develop allies to support your efforts is to share the changes you're making and the results you're getting. You may be surprised at who shows up to champion you and who might want to join you in this adventure. Even the simple act of sharing your successes is reinforcing—it can remind you why you're making the changes in the first place.

I would love to hear from you about how your journey goes and what happens along the way. You can contact me directly by email, at gerry@evolutionaryreboot.com or through my website at evolutionaryreboot.com, where you'll find additional helpful information to assist you on your journey, as well as information about my workshops and coaching programme, should you want additional support along the way.

I hope this book has been helpful. May you recognise the message of hope that underlies all the information I've presented here. Yes, you can fix your health by fixing your environment. Nothing is written in stone, and it's never too late to start.

I wish you well as you step into being the architect of your own healthy future.

RESOURCES

After reading this book, some of you may be interested in delving deeper into the information I introduced in the previous chapters. Others of you may find that you want some additional support as you begin to make the changes in your diet and environment that will help you to improve your health. From my own research over the past few years, I can tell you that there is a wealth of information available once you begin to look. The sheer volume can be daunting, and so, to give you a place to start, I've listed the following resources, many of which I referred to in the main text of the book.

Books

DIET AND NUTRITION
Death By Food Pyramid, Denise Minger (Primal Blueprint Publishing, 2013)

Epi-Paleo Rx, Jack Kruse, MD (Optimized Life PLC, 2013)

Food and Western Disease, Staffan Lindberg (Wiley-Blackwell, 2010)

Nutrition and Physical Degeneration, Weston A. Price (Benediction Classics, 2010)

Pure, White and Deadly, John Yudkin (Penguin Books, 1988, 2012)

The Paleo Manifesto, John Durant (Harmony, 2013)

The Statin Damage Crisis, Duane Graveline, MD, (Duane Graveline, MD, 2012)

LIGHT AND SLEEP
Great Sleep! Reduced Cancer!, Richard L. Hansler, PhD, (Richard L. Hansler, 2008)

Light in Shaping Life, Roeland Van Wijk (Meluna, Geldermalsen, 2014)

The Stanford Sleep Book, William C. Dement, MD, PhD, (2002)

ELECTROMAGNETISM AND GROUNDING
Earthing, Clinton Ober, Stephen T. Sinatra, MD, and Martin Zucker (Basic Health Publications, Inc., 2010)

Electromagnetism & Life, Robert O. Becker, MD, and Andrew A. Marino, PhD, JD (Cassandra Publishing, 2010)

The Body Electric, Robert O. Becker, MD, and Gary Selden (William Morrow, 1985)

WATER
The Fourth Phase of Water, Gerald H. Pollack (Ebner and Sons, 2013)

Your Body's Many Cries for Water, F. Batmanghelidj, MD (Global Health Solutions, 2008)

ATTITUDE AND SELF-HEALING
Mind Over Medicine, Lissa Rankin, MD (Hay House, Inc., 2013)

Websites & Other Publications

Reversing Disease for Optimal Health, Dr. Jack Kruse, jackkruse.com (blogs, webinars and forum/online community)

The More To Life Programme, www.moretolife.org (transformational trainings to support personal empowerment and shifting deep-seated beliefs)

What Doctor's Don't Tell You, www.wddty.com (a brilliant website and subscription magazine about leading-edge research on health, presented in non-geek language)

Continue Your Journey with Me

My hope is that you will find the information in this book useful for guiding you in identifying factors in your diet and environment that are likely to be contributing to chronic disease and early ageing, and that point to changes you can make that may greatly improve your health and wellbeing. That is the purpose of this book and of my workshops and coaching. I am a fellow traveller and an educator, not a doctor. I do not diagnose conditions or prescribe treatment—*you will need to take full responsibility for your health alongside your own health practitioner*, and this book is designed to empower you to do just that. What I *can* do is to help you to *diagnose your environment* and suggest ways to mitigate the elements that may be degrading your health and preventing healing.

I am also highly trained in methodologies that can help you break through the internal blocks that can trip you up along the way, so that you can put changes in place that are sustainable. You may find that you would like some additional support along the way to better understand the types of changes to make and to have help with working through some of the difficulties you may encounter. If you'd like to continue your journey with me, here are some options you might consider:

Participate in my flagship course, ReBoot Camp, which includes follow-up coaching support. You'll find details at evolutionaryreboot.com/offerings

Follow my blog posts at evolutionaryreboot.com/reboot-blog

Sign up for further notifications of blog posts and future events, at evolutionaryreboot.com

Sign up for a free telephone strategy session, at evolution aryreboot.com/strategy-session

ACKNOWLEDGMENTS

Although this book was only a few weeks in the writing, it was many decades in the preparation. This book is the culmination of knowledge and wisdom gathered over three different careers; from the influence of many teachers, mentors and healers; through the experience of finding my own way out of the downward health spiral; with the encouragement of friends and family; and with the guidance of a brilliant publishing team. To name everyone who helped to prepare me for getting this book to you would require another book altogether, but there are some people I specifically want to mention.

Two great teachers have influenced my thinking and, each in his own way, contributed to saving my life. The first is the late Dr. K. Bradford Brown who directly, through my many of our interactions, and indirectly, through the methodologies he designed, taught me how to identify and challenge limiting beliefs and to recognise the pearl of great price in any situation life presents. The second is Dr. Jack Kruse, who is more than a brilliant neurosurgeon. For more than four years he has been shining a light on the miraculous way the human body has been designed to function in concert with the environment we evolved within. He gives us a quantum lens through which we can begin to see the true causes of modern-day diseases and how to reverse them. At a personal level, he gave me a priceless gift: hope.

In that same vein, I'd like to acknowledge all the amazing researchers and health care practitioners—our modern-day Galileos—who have the courage to challenge conventional wisdom and entrenched belief systems, at great risk of public censure, in order to expand our understanding of how the human body works, deliver more effective treatments to patients, and pave the way for a new health-care paradigm. The model for the future of medicine will be built on their backs. It is their work that I have tried to distil into an understandable message so it can find its way into many hands through this book.

Without encouragement and support from many friends and family, I would not have had the courage to create my health education business, Evolutionary Reboot®, which became the platform for writing this book. My business took its name and shape in the kitchen of my sister-in-law, Bev, as she and I, along with my sister Ginger and my partner, brought the idea to life through our discussions. I also want to thank Sophie Sabbage for telling me over dinner one night (many wonderful things seem to emerge out of kitchen table conversations!) that I had to stop researching and write a book. Until that moment, it hadn't occurred to me that I had a story to tell. I didn't stop researching, but within a few weeks after that conversation, I was writing. A direct shot at the right time can make all the difference.

I also want to thank those who participated in my first workshops, for helping me find the non-geeky way to tell the evolutionary biology story and its great news about how we can change the course of our future and find our way to health and vitality. They helped me find my unique voice and they shaped what has become the flagship offering of my business.

I would have had no clue about how to write a book at all, never mind in just a few weeks, without Angela Lauria and her brilliant team at Difference Press. Being fiercely committed to helping others make a difference in the world made her programme the perfect match for me and for what I want this book to achieve. My developmental editor, Grace Kerina, has done a fabulous job of grasping what I'm trying to say and helping me say it better while preserving my voice. That is an art in itself.

Finally, I want to thank my partner, Hermione, for patiently listening to the first version of every chapter, for giving very helpful input about how my words were landing, and for handling the lion's share of managing builders, contractors, and keeping our home running in order to create the space and time for me to write. She may not have written the words, but she is my co-author in every other way.

ABOUT THE AUTHOR

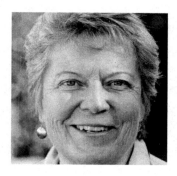

Dr. Gerilynn Moline is the owner of Evolutionary Reboot, an educational business offering seminars, workshops and coaching to the general public about the principles of evolutionary health and nutrition. She is also qualified as a Functional Diagnostics Nutrition-Practitioner. Her mission is to teach people how to reverse chronic illness and early ageing by realigning their environment to their biology as it was designed by evolution. This work was developed out of more than four years of in-depth research into leading-edge work that is being conducted in the fields of evolutionary health and quantum biology. Her research was driven by the desire to reverse her own chronic illness and to find a way to help others to do so.

Someone once described Gerry as the kind of person who puts her PhD in her back pocket and then gets down in the trenches with the people she works with. This was certainly true during her time as a US Air Force nurse, when her emphasis on patient care over military channels and procedures brought her accolades, along with occasionally landing her in hot water. It was also true during her 20-year research and academic career, where she was known for her "sticky note" lectures to students in her lab as she scribbled pictures on Post-It Notes to help them grasp complex concepts (while she taught them to have the courage of their convictions). And it has been true for the 18 years she's been training people to use deep transformational skills for shifting attitudes and making behavioural changes stick.

Gerry's varied careers have all been focused on one central purpose: making a difference in the lives of others. That's what gets her up in the morning. That and enjoying the English countryside with her partner and being barefoot in the grass as much as possible!

THANK YOU

Thank you for reading *Reboot Yourself!* I hope you found it helpful and learned a bit more about how our modern-day environment and diet are out of alignment with our biology and how you can begin to reverse those effects.

If you'd like help evaluating your environment and its possible impacts on your health, you can use the *Get Started Questionnaire*, which you can download for free from my website—evolutionaryreboot.com/get-started-questionnaire. The results of your survey, along with this book, will help you identify changes you can make to shift your health.

As a special bonus for readers of this book, if you want help working through or interpreting the *Get Started Questionnaire*, then I invite you to schedule a free 30-minute phone strategy session with me. You can schedule it through my website (evolutionaryreboot.com/strategy-session) or email me at gerry@evolutionaryreboot.com.

Finally, if you want additional support with identifying the changes you need to make to begin to turn your health around, or support in implementing and sticking to those changes, you'll find information about my seminars, workshops, and coaching at evolutionaryreboot.com/offerings

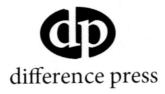

difference press

Difference Press offers solopreneurs, including life coaches, healers, consultants, and community leaders, a comprehensive solution to get their books written, published, and promoted. A boutique-style alternative to self-publishing, Difference Press boasts a fair and easy-to-understand profit structure, low-priced author copies, and author-friendly contract terms. Its founder, Dr. Angela Lauria, has been bringing to life the literary ventures of hundreds of authors-in-transformation since 1994.

LET'S START A MOVEMENT WITH YOUR MESSAGE

You've seen other people make a difference with a book. Now it's your turn. If you are ready to stop watching and start taking massive action. Reach out.

"Yes, I'm ready!"

In a market where hundreds of thousands books are published every year and are never heard from again, all participants of The Author Incubator have bestsellers that are actively changing lives and making a difference.

In less than two years we've created over 100 bestselling books in a row, 90% from first-time authors. As a result, our regular book programs are selling out in advance and we are selecting only the highest quality and highest potential applicants for our future programs.

Our program doesn't just teach you how to write a book—our team of coaches, developmental editors, copy editors, art directors, and marketing experts incubate you from book idea to published bestseller, ensuring that the book you create can actually make a difference in the world. We only work with the people who will use their book to get out there and make that difference.

If you have life-or world-changing ideas or services, a servant's heart, and the willingness to do what it REALLY takes to make a difference in the world with your book, go to http://theAuthorIncubator.com/apply to complete an application for the program today.

OTHER BOOKS BY DIFFERENCE PRESS

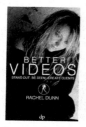

Better Videos: Stand out. Be Seen. Create Clients.

by Rachel Dunn

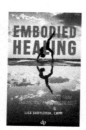

Embodied Healing: Using Yoga to Recover from Trauma and Extreme Stress

by Lisa Danylchuk

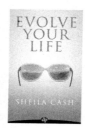

Evolve Your Life: Rethink Your Biggest Picture Through Conscious Evolution

by Sheila Cash

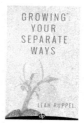

Growing Your Separate Ways: 8 Straight Steps to Separating with the Same Intention of Love and Respect You Had...

by Leah Ruppel

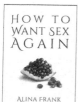

How to Want Sex Again: Rekindling Passion with EFT

by Alina Frank

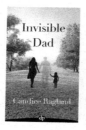

Invisible Dad: How to Heal as a Fatherless Daughter

by Candice Ragland

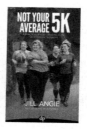

Not Your Average 5K: A Practical 8-Week Training Plan for Beginning Runners

by Jill Angie

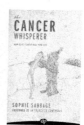

The Cancer Whisperer: How to Let Cancer Heal Your Life

by Sophie Sabbage

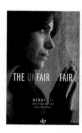

*The Unfair Affair:
How to Strengthen
and Save Your
Marriage, or Move
on with Confidence,
After Infidelity*

by Wendy Kay

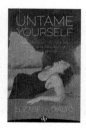

*Untame Yourself:
Reconnect to the
Lost Art, Power
and Freedom of
Being a Woman*

by Elizabeth DiAlto

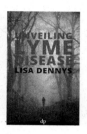

*Unveiling Lyme
Disease: Is
This What's
Behind Your
Chronic Illness?*

by Lisa Dennys

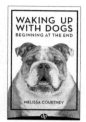

*Waking Up With
Dogs: Beginning
at the End*

by Melissa Courtney

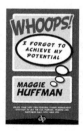

*Whoops! I Forgot
To Achieve My
Potential: Create
Your Very Own
Personal Change
Management
Strategy to Get the...*

by Maggie Huffman

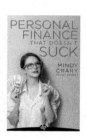

*Personal Finance
That Doesn't Suck: A
5-step Guide to Quit
Budgeting, Start
Wealth Building and
Get the Most from...*

by Mindy Crary

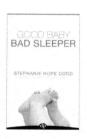

*Good Baby, Bad
Sleeper: Discover
Your Child's Sleep
Personality To
Finally Get the
Sleep You Need*

by Stephanie
Hope Dodd

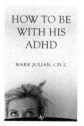

*How You Can Be
with His ADHD:
What You Can
Do To Rescue Your
Relationship When
Your Partner Has
Adult ADHD*

by Mark Julian

CPSIA information can be obtained
at www.ICGtesting.com
Printed in the USA
LVOW01s2020180716
496778LV00036BA/537/P